7.4.2

D1270515

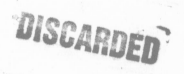

The Senseless Sacrifice:
A Black Paper on Medicine

The Senseless Sacrifice:
A Black Paper on Medicine

Heward Grafftey

McClelland and Stewart Limited/Toronto

0-7710-3500-4

The Canadian Publishers
McClelland and Stewart Limited
25 Hollinger Road, Toronto 374

Printed and bound in Canada

Contents

Acknowledgements

Over the past two years, in the United States and Canada, literally hundreds of students, doctors, medical-scientists, technicians, paramedical workers, interested citizens, hospital administrators, directors of public and private associations, government officials, journalists and others working in the news media have helped me in the preparation of this book. My mind goes back over scores of fascinating interviews and over the many written submissions which were so kindly afforded to me.

To list all those who gave so unselfishly of their time would be impossible. To say thank you is not enough, for without the many constructive suggestions, help and co-operation I received, this book would never have come to be.

However, two names must be mentioned. My thanks go to Paul Rush, Managing Editor of *Weekend* magazine, who helped in the organization of my material, and above all I thank Michael Baxendale, Director of Information Services, of the *Montreal Star*. His constructive criticism, suggestions, and untiring patience were invaluable, as he assisted me in every way imaginable.

It is my hope that this book, in some small way, will prove to be worthy of all the help and the many kindnesses I received during the two years spent in its writing.

Heward Grafftey
1971

To the Dead who should be living . . .
To the Sick who should be well . . .
This book is dedicated.

Introduction

North American Medical and Health Care Services are on the brink of total disaster. This is not scaremongering, but a statement of cold fact.

Canada, with the third highest standard of living in the world, ranks twentieth in doctor-population ratio. The United States is economically the world's richest country yet it ranks twenty-second in longevity and eighteenth in infant mortality.

In Canada, only half our doctors are now in the primary care field (general practitioners) compared to 67 per cent as recently as 1955.

In the U.S., there has been a 10 per cent decrease in the number of active physicians in relation to population since 1950. In the area of primary care, the number of general practitioners has dropped by one-third. It is now 50 per 100,000 population, as compared to the pre-Second World War figure of 135 per 100,000.

In the United States, 412,000 people in 155 counties do not have access to a physician at all. The distribution of doctors in cities is tragically out of balance. New York has an overall physician population ratio of 278 doctors per 100,000 residents. Yet in the poor and ghetto areas where help is most needed, the ratio is a disgraceful 10 doctors per 100,000 population.

Canada and the United States have the highest per capita ratios for uncontrolled heart disease in the world. Automobile accidents in North America continue to take a huge toll on life and health. The soaring number of mental and nervous breakdowns is alarming as is the soaring personal income of physicians. The physician is still rewarded in proportion to the malady of his patient. The longer it lasts, the more he makes. We still have no system to reward efficiency and penalize inefficiency and the self-regulating organizations of the profession including the A.M.A. and C.M.A. are in no hurry to change the status quo.

Reports of medical errors, doctor incompetence, and resultant human suffering run rampant in our everyday conversation. Yet for the average citizen, the "doctor" image still commands a certain degree of awe and forgiveness. In the meantime, medical care and services are deteriorating every day.

The urban poor and large rural populations have next to no services because of the poor distribution of facilities and manpower. We are lagging, inexcusably, behind in the whole area of preventative medicine. In both countries, doctors and hospitals are facing modern problems with outdated methods and absurdly old-fashioned attitudes. Neither the Canadian nor the American Medical Association have made any genuine effort toward progressive thinking. Predictably, neither Ottawa nor Washington has really begun to formulate the kind of national health policies which would give federal health services any true consistency and direction. Millions and millions of public and private dollars go down the drain, as hospitals continue to be managed by methods which would put a modern corporation into bankruptcy.

Waste and duplication plague our system. It is not the sole fault of the doctors, but they no longer enjoy the blind confidence they received in past years. They now find themselves under the eye of an increasingly critical and questioning public. Recently, Senator Abraham Ribicoff chaired in Washington a sub-committee on executive reorganization dealing with medical care in the United States. The findings were so alarming that they prompted the following words from then Secretary of Health, Education and Welfare, Robert H. Finch: "This nation is faced with a breakdown in the delivery of health services unless immediate and concerted action is taken by government and the private sector."

Since the turn of the century, we have seen a tremendous advance in the art of medicine and medical technology. Concurrently, public expectations have soared. In so many ways, progress has been the hallmark of the North American dream. The state of contemporary medical services is turning that dream into a nightmare. Too many people who desperately need care are not getting it. Too many people who should be living are dead.

1
Yesterday and Tomorrow

Every day lives are sacrificed at the altar of the non-system.

Suppose you come to a town where the people are starving and you want to help them? It happens that you are wealthy, that you have enough money for every person in town. What do you do? Of course, you give them all money. But it doesn't do any good for there's no food available for them to buy – and they keep on starving.

Absurd? Yes. But the parallel is frighteningly close to the present organization of medical services in North America – money has been voted for and put into people's pockets for services that just aren't there. To avoid total breakdown, we need radical change and reform. The "non-system" must go.

In medicine we have now taken the first steps in genetic engineering. The centuries-old dream of re-growing limbs has been revived. An almost perfect test to screen blood serum against hepatitis infection has been developed. Evidence that viruses may cause arthritis and other inflammatory diseases has opened the way to the development of an arthritis vaccine. All these are causes for rejoicing. Yet other medical discoveries of decades ago are still not helping the "majority" of North Americans. Our shocking delivery system has made sure of that. In most of the inner cores of large cities and outlying areas in North America, care and treatment are thirty to forty years behind the times. Every day lives are sacrificed at the altar of the "non-system," because scant attention has been paid to delivering "services to people." Under present conditions, the achievements of today might never reach the majority of North Americans.

Right now things are so bad that many feel we are losing the battle against disease which, for so long, we seemed to be winning. Heart disease, lung cancer, and chronic respiratory illness have caused overall mortality rates to creep up again after one hundred and fifty years of sharp decline.

The modern watershed in medical progress was the Second World War. Even though it was responsible for millions of deaths, it also paved the way for great breakthroughs in medicine, and ultimately the saving of millions of lives. Before the Second World War, scientific findings and techniques were recognized by all to be an increasingly significant aspect of modern society, but few had first-hand contact with scientific findings and even fewer had any real appreciation of science's nature and achievement. Knowledge was largely reserved for a small minority of academic people and it touched the lives of most men only indirectly through its influence on technology – with especial reference to transportation, communications and medical practice. The war brought science into government, and into the techniques of combat. It also brought politics, economics and social responsibility into science in a way which could only be beneficial to all. The consequence of these revolutionary advances now surround us on all sides. As historian Carroll Quigley points out, they "are obvious, even to the most uncomprehending, in television and electronics, in biology and medical science, in space exploration, in automation of credit, billing, payroll and personnel practices, in atomic energy and above all in the constant threat of nuclear incineration."

It is the medical advances which are our main present concern. For example, one of the greatest victories of science in the war was the treatment of the wounded. Ninety-seven per cent of the casualties who reached the front-line dressing stations were saved, a figure which had never been approached in earlier wars. The techniques which made this possible, involving blood transfusions, surgical techniques, and anti-bodies have all been continued and amplified in the post-war world, although the destruction of man's natural environment by the further irresponsible development of technology has created new causes of death by advancing cancer, disintegrating circulatory systems, and increasing mental breakdowns.

Nevertheless, great progress has still been made and fantastic scientific advances have been paralleled by equally drastic changes in social attitudes. If the development of new medical techniques is one side of the coin, the other side of the same coin has been the emergence of an increasingly sensitive social conscience.

And there's the rub. The new scientific breakthroughs in medicine, combined with heightened demand by a consumer society for medical goods and services – and the undertaking by government to provide and underwrite these services – have caused costs to climb higher than anyone could have foreseen.

Both in Canada and the United States billions of public dollars have been put into citizen's pockets in the form of income supplementation to buy services which are either non-existent, or which governments have done next to nothing to improve or increase. In the United States, Medicare and Medicaid, the government-financed programmes for paying the medical expenses of the aged and the poor, now account for $1 out of every $5 spent on medical services. In Canada the total health service expenditures, including both private and public, have risen from about $1.75 billions in 1960 to about $4.2 billions in 1968.

It is not just the schemes designed to pay the doctor's bills that cost the money. The new artifacts of medicine are often as complex and impressive as those on that more visible frontier of technology – space. In the same way as space hardware, the new devices are usually expensive. A linear accelerator is valued at $200,000; a new cyclotron would cost about $300,000; and the neurosurgery suite at Mount Zion hospital in San Francisco cost $200,000.

Once the equipment is procured, however, the costs have just begun. Mt. Sinai in New York is spending an estimated $550,000 annually to maintain and operate its hyperbaric chamber, a high-pressure chamber used in testing for brain malfunction. The widely-used kidney machine costs an average $15,000 annually per patient in upkeep of materials and staff. Patients are unable to cover expenses on such a scale themselves, and with hospital endowments and federal subsidies failing to keep pace, hospitals are hard-pressed for funds to operate these advanced facilities. Both in rural areas and in the poverty areas of our cities, patients die each year for lack of treatment that is within technical, but not financial reach.

Glaring problems now facing United Kingdom and North American medical and health care services could be summed up under four general headings: shortages, inequitable distribution, organizational deficiency, and lack of money.

Taken together these are conditions which cry out for reform. The physician himself has a useful way of making the distinction we are after. He distinguishes between diseases arising from local causes or disturbances, and those that can be called "systematic." Systematic diseases are traced to some fundamental disability of the organism as a whole, so that its entire principle of operation is being interfered with. To be effective, the corrective treatment must be as profound as the scope of the disorder. Social systems can be spoken of in the same way, and so can the state of our medical and health services. Medieval kingship was incapable of providing the fiscal base required by government in industrial societies. Similarly, the traditional methods

3

of organizing our doctors and distributing health services are inadequate for coping with the new and increasing demands of contemporary society. North Americans at every level of society are being badly served by the obsolete, overstrained medical system that has grown up around them in a helter-skelter fashion, with no real attempt to accommodate the changing technology, expanding population, rising costs, or our rising expectations. The fact that a shortage of doctors does exist, and is going to continue to exist, is but one of the many symptoms of the general malaise.

The management of medical and health care has become too important to leave to doctors, who are, after all, not managers to begin with. The medical profession must find ways to improve its productivity and some of these ways may have to be forced upon it. The financial distortions, the inequities and the managerial redundancies in our medical and health care system are of the kind that society cannot be expected to tolerate for long. To repeat my earlier statements – the time has come for radical change and the non-system must go. By examining some of the most glaring defects of that "system" as it exists today, let us discover where change is most desperately needed.

2
Our Non-Existent Emergency Services

We called the police three times before they sent an ambulance. – ARNOLD DEACON, CANADIAN FARMER

It was a sunny day on Friday, August 21, 1964, when I left my Ottawa apartment around 7 a.m., to board an east-bound Canadian Pacific Railway train for Montreal. About the same time as the train pulled out of Ottawa's Union Station, Basil Czopyk was driving his truck full of rocks toward Leonard, Ontario, a small village on the C.P. rail line between Ottawa and Montreal. Czopyk usually stopped for coffee at Leonard. From time to time he boasted how he raced and beat the early morning train over the rail intersection in the middle of this quiet hamlet. This particular Friday morning he wasn't going to make it. My train picked up speed as it left the outskirts of Ottawa. Twenty minutes after departure we were hitting around seventy miles per hour. I had taken a chair in the dining car to eat breakfast and read the newspaper. Then it happened!

The car began to pitch and lunge. People and furniture were thrown everywhere. Orange and yellow flames enveloped the windows. I was thrown the length of the car with piles of other diners. Finally the car came to a crashing halt at an acute angle. I scrambled out and jumped on to the gravel rail bed. It was hard, at first, to understand just what had happened. In front of me was the wreckage of a truck amidst a pile of stones. Czopyk had driven into the middle of the train. He was killed instantly. The engine and front cars continued on. The car he hit left the tracks going end over end like a football before falling on its side in a nearby field. Those in the dining car, including myself, and in one more car at the rear of the train, were fortunate. Automatic brakes went on, and while many were shaken up as these two cars ripped up a hundred yards of track, many injuries were prevented and lives saved. But the car that was hit lay on its side near an old farm shed. I could hear the screams and moans that issued from its interior.

Sliding down the embankment to the scene, I could see what had happened. As the car spun in mid-air, many were tossed through broken windows, then the car rolled over and crushed them. It was difficult to tell who was dead and who was injured. A stunned train-man attempted to set up communications with some equipment which he attached to the tracks. I ran to a nearby farmhouse and on an old crank phone told the operator of the accident, asking for ambulances. Forty minutes later, a country doctor arrived. Helicop-ters from the news media hovered over the scene of the tragedy. Finally, more than one hour after the accident, one privately-owned ambulance appeared.

I don't know when the last victim was removed, but many seri-ously injured passengers still lay in the field more than two hours after the crash. And we were not miles away from civilization in some isolated wilderness, but only twenty minutes from our nation's capi-tal. The final toll: eight dead and more than twenty seriously injured.

In the mid-winter of 1970, Arnold Deacon and his twenty-year-old daughter, Monica, heard a loud boom. Monica looked out the win-dow of the kitchen in her Waterville, Quebec, home near the Quebec/ Vermont border. A bus had crashed off a nearby bridge. After spot-ting the mangled wreckage of the bus and people strewn in the snow on the river bed, the Deacons called the police then immediately took several blankets to comfort the injured while awaiting the ambul-ances. Arnold Deacon later said that he and his daughter called the police three times before ambulances arrived on the scene. The police told him they couldn't help because it wasn't in their area of cover-age. Twenty-two of the passengers had been injured, several critically. When help finally arrived, it was too late for 17-year-old Carol Dupuis of Beebe. She was already dead.

In a rural area of Quebec, a traffic victim lay in the snow in mid-winter. The investigating police officer wasn't certain in which ambu-lance region the accident had taken place, so he called two ambulances to make sure – one from each adjacent area. Forty minutes later, one ambulance arrived; but before the operator could load the victim aboard, the second was at the scene. The police officer soon had to rule over the ugly argument which arose between the operators, both of whom claimed a right to the victim.

The above are only three examples – but such tragedies occur with horrifying frequency. Somewhere along the line we have mixed up our priorities. Generally speaking, proper emergency services are a community responsibility which, admittedly, require the assistance and understanding of senior governments. When we are faced with property damage, police are at the scene of a crime in no time at all. Alarms bring fire engines, trained personnel and expensive equipment speeding to a fire. Yet when it comes to the question of physical injury or illness, we allow our fellow man to suffer and sometimes to die, after lying exposed to the elements under the morbid gaze of the curious. Why? The answer to this reveals one of the disgraceful deficiencies in our society.

Let us ask ourselves a few basic questions:

If I am seriously injured or fall seriously ill, would my transportation to hospital be organized in a manner most conducive to my recovery?

If I arrived at hospital, unconscious and unidentified, would I receive the best possible life-saving treatment? Would there be properly trained personnel available to treat me?

Are there the necessary facilities in my hospital to admit me to a resuscitation room immediately, or would "red tape" kill me?

Would there be sufficient blood and plasma substitutes available, and would experienced personnel be on duty to conduct the necessary resuscitation and investigations where required?

Would emergency staff realize that perhaps I shouldn't be moved from my stretcher or be given an anesthetic which might cause death as a result of my degree of shock?

Would someone be on hand immediately to take the necessary X-Ray pictures and tests, and could the stretcher be placed on the X-Ray table without moving me off it?

Would the operating room staff personnel be ready to go into immediate action within ten minutes, or would I die as they got ready?

Generally speaking there's only one answer to most of these questions. It is "No."

The vast majority of North America's community ambulance services are hit-and-miss affairs, based on a "haul for hire" operation. Both in our urban and rural areas, funeral directors often run the local ambulance service. Reports indicate that the majority of these operators would like to get out of the ambulance business simply because they lose money on it. Many continue the work reluctantly, only because there would be a howl of local public indignation if they pulled out of this much-needed community emergency service. It is also true that, in certain instances, private ambulance operators have refused to transport accident victims or the seriously ill until payment has been guaranteed. Some justify this by saying that they collect only about forty per cent of their bills (interestingly enough, only a very few public or private medical plans cover ambulance costs). And there are further problems. Because of poor communications equipment and organization, or none, most of these privately-owned vehicles arrive at the scene of accidents, or to pick up the seriously ill, too late. This is only part of the story. Far too often the personnel operating ambulance vehicles are in no way trained to handle or deal with the sick or injured. Also, the vehicles, in many instances hearses, hurriedly converted to ambulance service, are in no way designed or equipped to play their proper part in transporting and treating the people. Dr. Campbell Gardner, a surgeon at the Montreal General Hospital, reported the following: "I was telephoned about transporting an accident victim to the hospital and I suggested that he should have an adequate supply of blood, presuming that this would be commenced before starting and continued on the way. To my horror, the patient arrived at the hospital, complete with four unopened bottles of blood in the ambulance."

Wilder Penfield, the famed neurosurgeon at the Montreal Neurological Institute, noted that inexperienced handling of back injury patients often resulted in severed spinal chords and lifetime paraplegia. Other accident surgeons have reported alarming numbers of unnecessary deaths because of shock resulting from severe fractures which have not been properly splinted or even splinted at all.

Recently, Penfield pointed out to me how well co-ordinated ambulance dispatch systems were handled in Russia, both at Leningrad's and Moscow's centres for Traumatology. We would do well to take heed. Proper communications enable ambulances to be dispatched from central dispatch centres and directed to proper treatment centres. While sometimes unnecessary speed is employed in driving, the personnel are extremely well-trained, and Moscow and Leningrad have one of the world's best ambulance services.

Certainly, however, excessive speed in ambulances constitutes yet another serious hazard and it doesn't only happen in Russia. One of my first law cases, as a student, involved an accident victim who had broken a leg. He had been seriously injured as the speeding ambulance transporting him to hospital crashed at a city intersection. The judge questioned whether a broken leg required high speed transportation. In May of 1970, Michel Brière, a twenty-year-old centre with the Pittsburg Penguins of the National Hockey League, was being transported to hospital in Montreal by ambulance after he had been injured in a car accident. Speeding to Montreal, the ambulance itself was involved in a crash, killing 18-year-old Raymond Perrault of Malartic, Quebec. Brière, himself, died a year later, never having regained consciousness.

To combat this kind of tragedy, Dr. Basil C. MacLean, Commissioner, City of New York, Department of Hospitals, in 1955 reported on a pilot study at King's County Hospital from October 1, 1953 to August 1, 1954. All sirens were removed from ambulances and other departmental vehicles and all operators were given strict orders to obey normal traffic regulations. Accidents were cut in half.

In the field of emergency services, obsolete methods die hard and rarely does the public benefit from progressive emergency technology. The British Army Medical Corps adopted the use of traction splints for compound fractured femurs in 1917. This reduced the mortality from such injuries from 80 per cent to 20 per cent. A mortality rate of over 50 per cent for penetrating wounds treated by general surgeons in the First World War was reduced by Harvard's Harvey Cushing to 28 per cent. This figure was further reduced to approximately 15 per cent in the Second World War and 7.8 per cent in Korea. Vietnam figures are even lower. Fast transportation from the front lines through evacuation centres, often using helicopters, to neurosurgical units is largely responsible for such improvements. Yet in civilian life we haven't even begun to apply lessons that have long been in use by the military in theatres of war.

It is unrealistic to lay sole blame on the private ambulance operators and attendants in Canada and the United States. Basically, the public is not aware of the situation – the system takes care of that. Different levels of government disclaim all financial or moral responsibility.

With a few notable exceptions which we will examine later, we find no public standards for ambulance design and equipment, no public standards relating to emergency treatment personnel, communications, and the reorganization, staffing, and equipping of emergency units in hospitals. The medical profession has persistently avoided contact with ambulance services. Thus, private services rarely, if ever, obtained training to upgrade their treatment facilities. Even if they had, it is questionable whether the jealousy of the medical profession would have allowed ambulance attendants to "practice doctoring" by even applying splints or stopping bleeding. The Emergency Health

9

Services Division of the Ontario Hospital Service Commission recently started training casualty care attendants, thus initiating a new paramedical discipline. Tragically but predictably, the medical profession for the most part has tended to reject this new concept. Surely it is now time for the profession to admit the inability of doctors to be at all roadside or sick-bed casualties. The facts of life must be accepted. Public authorities, working with the medical profession, must train people to take the doctor's place. Doctors should be reluctant to waste their energies in destructive criticism of a system organized by government when, as a professional group, they are too indifferent, too busy, or too lazy to do anything about it. The present chaos in North American emergency services cannot continue. They require immediate upgrading, direction, organization, and co-ordination, and the public should expect and demand no less. The medical profession has a great opportunity to extend and improve its services to society by supporting this new philosophy and by volunteering its aid, but judging by its present attitudes the likelihood of this occurring is virtually non-existent.

There is only one possible conclusion to this chapter. Emergency services in North America are in a mess. Far too many North Americans have died or have been permanently incapacitated because we have failed to apply proven technological data and medical facts to the fundamental principles of emergency treatment.

3
Emergency Services – Part 2

*Montreal provides one of the most imaginative ambu-
lance services in the world, probably because not too long
ago, it had one of the worst.*

Perhaps the hardest truth to accept about medical emergency services
is that there is virtually no excuse for them being as bad as they are.
The few specific exceptions to the overall chaos show just how far
short of the optimum general conditions are.

In New York City, there are twenty city-run hospitals which operate their own ambulances. The procedure, at the scene of an accident,
is to get to a phone as quickly as possible and tell the police. The
police don't stall – they do two things. First, they notify the hospital
nearest to the scene of the accident which sends an ambulance. Second, they come to the scene themselves. All police operators know
which city-run hospital is closest to the area the call came from. If for
some reason the police number is unavailable, a call to the telephone
operator sets the same procedure in motion.

An incident in 1968 at New York's Columbia Presbyterian Medical Centre graphically points up the speed of the city's ambulance
procedure. A man was walking by the Medical Centre, a private
hospital, when he fell and broke his leg. By the time the nurses inside
Columbia Presbyterian were able to get a stretcher and move outside,
an ambulance had already pulled up from one of the city hospitals.

Montreal provides one of the most imaginative ambulance services in the world, probably because not too long ago, it had one of
the worst. Media and public indignation became so vociferous that
City Hall was shamed into action.

I remember witnessing a car hit a tree in mid-town Montreal
when I was in high school. Three people received severe multiple
injuries. They writhed in agony before my eyes. It took over forty-five
minutes for a private ambulance to arrive. The emergency ward of
one of the city's largest hospitals, the Royal Victoria, was no more
than a five-minute walk away from the accident. I remember the
anger and despair I felt at that scene.

Today, a fleet of over thirty police-ambulances gives the city around-the-clock coverage – seven days a week. The service takes care of people who are sick, or who are injured on the street or in public places. Exceptions are made for extreme home cases or for the urgent need of oxygen. The police-ambulance service is equipped with station-wagon type vehicles which are completely equipped. Constables assigned to the function of ambulance-man receive special advanced first-aid training, and while cruising throughout the city in these station-wagon ambulances, they also attend to their police duties.

In 1963, a statistical and efficiency review of the Montreal service was established. Findings showed that the average time for an ambulance to reach an accident scene after a call was received at the Police Emergency Communications Centre, amounted to 2.4 minutes, as compared to the average 9.6 minutes for private ambulances. The citizens are grateful.

Dorval, a suburb of Montreal, is served in the same fashion. Carol Rogerson and her husband George, of The Bolton Pass, Quebec, were visiting their daughter in Dorval in January, 1970, when Mrs. Rogerson fell to the floor with a stroke. Mr. Rogerson rushed to call the police.

"A cruiser ambulance arrived in three or four minutes," he told me. "They brought oxygen with them and they knew what to do. Carol was in the Lachine General Hospital in less than 20 minutes.

Doctors said that any delays could have been fatal."

Obviously, Mrs. Rogerson was one of the lucky ones.

Unfortunately, New York and Montreal, the two largest cities in their respective countries, are exceptions to the general North American rule. In the United States and Canada nothing in the medical and health fields varies more than the effectiveness, speed and standard of ambulance service from city to city and from area to area.

Canadian emergency communications are for the most part so primitive that they deserve open ridicule. For years, city taxis in North America have been equipped with two-way radios. Yet, most of our ambulances have no communications equipment. Early observation and documentation are vital in the treatment of accident victims. Fast information relayed by trained ambulance personnel to the emergency wards of hospitals, amongst other things, saves time and leads to a proper and fast diagnosis by the attending doctor.

What happens when an emergency patient finally arrives at an emergency centre? Medical technology has made spectacular advances in the past few decades, but this has had little effect on methods of emergency treatment. The indictment continues from the tragedy of our ambulance services to the tragedy of our treatment centres. The seriously ill or injured arrive at hospitals where emergency units are often combined with out-patient departments. This is especially true in the hard-core poverty areas of large city hospitals where emergency services are of extreme importance. Here those desperately needing medical attention crowd into out-patient departments which are also the hospital emergency units. They are often badly designed and laid out and they frequently lack fundamental emergency equipment. Worse, when they do have it, it is not unusual to find that nobody around can operate it. Almost as a general rule, untrained personnel subject accident victims to unnecessary and dangerous movement between the time they reach emergency units, go through preliminary examinations, X-Rays, and finally reach the operating theatre. Sometimes hours are wasted through red tape. Badly injured accident victims are X-Rayed and go through tests, unattended by qualified and trained help.

In the spring of 1970, I attended many of the sessions in Ottawa of the Ontario Medical Association. The sessions devoted to emergency services revealed an appalling fact: These services were often in frightful disarray and the Association, to its credit, openly admitted it.

It took a coroner's jury, in May of 1970, in Toronto, to finally rule that patients admitted to hospital emergency departments with head injuries should not be left unattended until a complete diagnosis has been carried out. The jury also urged the administration board of Toronto Western Hospital to adopt definite rules covering patients admitted to the emergency department. The jury made its recommendations after finding that William Singleton, 55, may have received severe head injuries after falling out of a stretcher in the hospital. Mr. Singleton had injured his head on March 24 when he fell down a flight of stairs in his home. After being admitted to emergency, attendants said he showed symptoms of a concussion and had dried blood on the back of his head. An attending doctor said she put up the side railings of Mr. Singleton's stretcher and left him alone for a few minutes. Two minutes later, she glanced back and saw him lying on the floor in convulsions. Mr. Singleton was unconscious and surgery was performed to remove two blood clots from his brain. He died the following day. Doctors said they could not tell coroner Dr. Elie Cass whether Mr.

Singleton died from injuries received from falling down stairs or from later falling from the stretcher.

Earlier in 1970, another coroner's jury decided the death of a Toronto man intent on suicide may very well have been due to Toronto East General Hospital's failure to treat him for the poison he had swallowed. The five-member jury, investigating the death of Douglas Wardrope, 31, strongly recommended that emergency ward admission reports be standardized to avoid the kind of confusion which surrounded the death of Mr. Wardrope. He was brought to the hospital after swallowing as much as 10 ounces of gas-line antifreeze which contains 97 per cent deadly methyl alcohol. He was physically healthy but apparently very depressed and suicidal when emergency ward Dr. David Stephen examined him. Dr. Stephen said it was not made clear to him the patient had consumed the poison, although the can of antifreeze had been brought to the hospital with him. The doctor recommended psychiatric treatment. The first psychiatric ward doctor to examine him said he was unable to clearly read the handwritten, carbon copy of the admittance report and believed Mr. Wardrope when he said he had consumed gasoline, not gas-line anti-freeze. The patient entered a deep coma which was not attributed to the poison he had taken and was not treated. He died twelve hours later. The coroner told the jury there had been a series of misunderstandings and breakdowns of communication at the hospital in this case, and possible lack of acceptance of responsibility for proper treatment by the doctors was involved. Dr. E. G. Cross, physician-in-chief at the hospital, told the jury the basic responsibility for treatment lay with the doctor who first admitted a patient, but said there had been a "breakdown in procedures." The jury also recommended to the chief coroner of Ontario that the time between a death and an inquest be as short as possible to enable witnesses to give as clear a report as possible.

Another irony of ironies is the fact that ambulances arriving at Canadian hospitals, even when the hospitals have been notified, invariably find no doctor on duty to administer emergency treatment. From Friday afternoons to Monday mornings is the peak time for traffic injuries yet, incredibly, emergency personnel and doctors are often "away for the weekend." Planned staffing of emergency wards is imperative. It is also widely resisted by many hospitals and doctors.

Dr. I. S. Raudin of the American College of Surgeons' Committee on Trauma has said, "It is our opinion that the worst care of patients at present, in many areas of our country, is in the field of trauma [shock]. This is true not only of the care received at the site of the accident, but also of the transportation of the injured and of the initial care received in the receiving wards of many hospitals."

One of the first elementary rules of first-aid is to "treat for shock." Emergency treatment frequently requires little more than first-aid training. Yet only Queen's Medical School in Kingston, Ontario, of all Canada's medical schools, currently gives anything like an adequate course to students in emergency and first-aid treatment. The great percentage of Canadian and u.s. medical students receive no first-aid emergency training at all. Dr. Robert Kennedy, one of the most skilful of all traumatic surgeons summarized today's situation extremely well: "There has been no organized effort to train the medical profession in first-aid. The medical schools which give any instruction in this subject are a rare exception. The result is that the average medical student, on receiving his degree, knows less about it than a first-class boy scout. If he takes an internship in a hospital with an ambulance service, if he becomes an industrial, mine, railroad, or police surgeon, he may become interested. But in most instances these activities are soon shunted to the sideline and his interest wanes. The rank and file of the profession consider the subject outside their field or are not aware of its extent and importance. The prime movers in first-aid instruction have, therefore, come from the lay public, aided by an occasional physician. Improved forms of treatment are adopted by the medical profession, but may not be incorporated in first-aid books for years, because the profession did not know how to place them before a layman practically. In other instances, first-aid workers have devised improved methods which have not been adopted generally by the medical profession because of lack of close contact with the work. Much is to be gained in the care of the injured by closer cooperation between these two groups to their mutual advantage."

Dr. Kennedy said this thirty-four years ago. It remains an accurate assessment of today's conditions.

Even if a patient in severe shock arrives at the hospital alive, another grim statistic further narrows his survival chances. Fewer than one per cent of Canadian and American hospitals are set up to give shock treatment around the clock.

Treatment of accident victims is also hindered by the question of public liability. Doctors and laymen alike sometimes refuse to help for fear of being sued by a victim who feels the helper actually aggra-

15

vated injury, or by next of kin, who claim the helper contributed to death.

Officials of the Canadian Medical Association insist this is a myth, stating that, to their knowledge, there have been no successful suits of this kind. Nonetheless, the province of Alberta found it necessary to pass a "Good Samaritan Act" protecting all those, laymen and doctors alike, from public liability, who render help in good faith to accident victims.

Of course, a major problem in regard to emergency treatment lies in our medical schools.

As already noted, Queen's University in Kingston is the only Canadian medical school where anything like an adequate emergency training course is given to students. The same situation exists throughout the United States' medical schools, with only a few exceptions. One involves the University of Kansas School of Medicine where Dr. Roger L. Youmans, Director of Emergency Services, University of Kansas Medical Center, and Dr. Richard A. Brose, Assistant Professor of Preventative Medicine and Community Health, are largely responsible for progress at this school.

The whole approach of the Kansas Medical Faculty to emergency training rests on the assumption that in emergency situations, the first hour of treatment can mean the difference between life and death.

At Kansas, fourth-year students now undergo a two-week clerkship which includes formal daily lecture discussions on a variety of practical emergency-care problems. They are also assigned to emergency departments on a twenty-four-hour-per-day basis.

Emergency medical technicians are also trained at the University in correct methods of caring for accident victims both at the scene and *en route* to hospital.

The University of Kansas and Queen's University show what can be done in the field but until other medical schools follow their lead, we cannot expect the medical profession to play any significant role in first-aid and emergency treatment.

In a way this lack of communication illustrates a classic truism of medical practice: positive findings are rarely communicated, let alone applied.

In the past thirty years Dr. Kennedy, as Director of the American College of Surgeon's Committee on Traumas field programme, initiated many constructive programmes. His manual entitled, *Emergency Care of the Sick and Injured* was distributed to communities all over

16

North America, as was his *Standards for Emergency Departments in Hospitals.* In 1967 the Committee also adopted *Standards for Emergency Ambulance Services.* Dr. Kennedy and his staff personally surveyed more than one hundred and fifty ambulance services in the United States and Canada and from their investigations a brilliant model ordinance on ambulance service was developed. More than five years have now passed since Kennedy made his recommendations and only a handful of communities have even begun to consider applying them. For the most part, they are either unknown to the communities or completely ignored by those responsible to the people for emergency services. The conclusion is obvious: Until publicly developed standards are enforced by public officials in the interest of society, little or no progress will be made.

While it is felt by most authorities that action on the community level is the answer, progress is almost non-existent.

Dr. Paul E. Paetow, of Hoboken, New Jersey, recently wrote, "While everyone agrees that emergency care of the injured and critically ill must be a community responsibility, making this concept work often proves to be a frustrating experience."

Dr. Harold Elliott of Como, Quebec, not only shares Paetow's views but has acted on them. Dr. Elliott was the Neurosurgeon in Chief of the Montreal General Hospital. Working long frustrating hours, night after night, over crushed heads which had been smashed against car corner posts and projected through windshields, he decided to try to get to the root causes of highway and automobile deaths and injuries. In 1966, with federal assistance, Elliott started a research project on a network of roads in the Ottawa area in order to determine why people were getting into accidents, and, once in them, what was killing or injuring drivers and passengers. Medical students formed part of the team investigating accidents in his project. They rode in ambulances and witnessed at first hand the performance of emergency operations.

Elliott was angered at the incredible disorganization of the community emergency response system. In one of the most important recommendations in his report to Ottawa, he stated emphatically, "It is no longer good enough for hospitals to boast about their individual performances once patients are admitted to their doors." "Hospitals," Elliott emphasizes, "must accept responsibilities outside their doors, and accept at least partial responsibility for accident rates in

17

their community and for the efficient response of proper emergency treatment facilities once accidents or sudden illness occurs."

The ultimate objectives of any emergency care system must be, primarily, twenty-four-hour availability of services for all residents and visitors in a community who require it. If every North American community measured its emergency services against such a basic set of requirements, the general results would be shocked disbelief. Whether or not this would lead to action is yet another thing.

Properly constructed and equipped vehicles are fundamental considerations in any modern emergency response system. Yet, frequently vehicles in use are not primarily designed as ambulances. Design and equipment take on increasing importance when we consider loading and unloading the patient, the smoothness of the ride, and the fact that trained personnel can work *en route* and require plenty of space and good light. Some progressive programmes even take into account the best colours for the interior of the vehicle. Ambulances and equipment should, but hardly ever do, meet such elementary standards as configuration of the patient compartment of each type of ambulance, common colour and identification lights, signs and horns for easy recognition by the public, standardization of items such as cots, litters, oxygen, and equipment to facilitate interchange between vehicles, and the development of an exchange system between treatment facilities and ambulances.

Ambulances are not the only consideration. Some cities, including Chicago, have provided for helicopter transport. Cook County Hospital has a special burn treatment unit. During a virtually complete motor-vehicle standstill following a snow storm in early 1967, a five-year-old girl, Robin Dean, severely burned in her home when her dress caught fire, was transferred to the Cook County burn unit from another hospital by helicopter after the physicians decided that the severe burns to 65 per cent of her body could only be treated in the special burn unit. Little Robin Dean died on March 16, 1967, after a five-week fight for life.

In October 1967, the Robin Dean Heliport was dedicated by Richard Ogilvie, now Governor of Illinois. It is directly across the street from the main entrance to Cook County hospital. The Chicago Fire Department has obtained two helicopters equipped to pick up any emergency patient anywhere in Chicago and the surrounding highways for both secondary and, more importantly, primary emergency helicopter transport.

Helicopters should be used far more frequently for primary transport of the sick and injured, certainly in built-up areas where road traffic conditions are increasingly congested. Picking up the injured on busy expressways, thruways and turnpikes should be a future use for the helicopter. Such use, though, must be facilitated by an organized approach by all authorities in providing proper and sensible landing facilities on traffic arteries. Seeing a tied-up ambulance carrying a seriously injured person on a city expressway in rush-hour traffic must become a thing of the past.

When considering emergency transport, let us recall the Montreal police ambulance service. There is no reason why the police ambulance principle should not be extended to other cities, small towns, villages, and rural areas. Properly constructed and equipped vehicles manned by competent personnel should always be included in such plans. The most frequent argument against this concept is that police should stick to police work. Yet police are most often the first to arrive at the scene of an accident. Villages and small towns should make sure at least one of their police cars is so converted and equipped and that police officers have advanced paramedical emergency training. Certainly, the same applies to provincial police in Canada, and state troopers in the United States. In Canadian provinces where the federal Mounted Police operate, they too could man police ambulances. Of course, not all police cars should be ambulances; but such cars should be regularly placed and on patrol on freeways, expressways, turnpikes, autoroutes, and inter-state highways.

One of the earliest conclusions reached in Ontario on the subject of casualty attendants was that some means must be found for assuring competent regular employees of full-time ambulance or emergency service and the opportunity of making a career of emergency paramedical work. This means those involved could initially be trained to "ride the ambulances." After further advanced training they would move into the emergency units in hospitals and even into the emergency operation theatres.

When it is seen what can be done with some imagination and organizational know-how, North Americans have reason to look with shocked disbelief at the general level of our emergency and first-aid training facilities.

On Friday, December 15, 1967, during the 5 p.m. rush hour, a 1,750 ft. span of the Silver Bridge across the Ohio River between Gallipolis, Ohio, and Point Pleasant, West Virginia, suddenly collapsed. What happened next tells something of the importance of efficient communications in disaster situations.

The traffic on the east-bound lane was heavy, and on the west-bound lane bumper-to-bumper. The Ohio was fifty feet deep at this point. The suddenness of the catastrophe was shown by the fact that pigeons which roost on the bridge were found trapped in the super-structure. Within minutes, dozens of observers called the telephone company which in turn alerted the appointment desk at the Holzer Hospital and Clinic, the police, and fire departments.

At the Holzer Hospital, many of the staff were completing their work day. The chief of staff immediately put the disaster plan in motion and had members of the staff who had left called back. Then the telephone system broke down completely. It remained out of order for approximately fifteen to twenty minutes.

The news of the disaster had hit the media so fast that the local telephone system was almost immediately overloaded. As soon as the telephone company's supervisory personnel arrived at its office, they instituted a load-control mechanism which allowed service to a select list of designated emergency personnel, hospital, police, and fire departments. Although this service continued, it was retarded by incoming calls for approximately two hours.

Donald M. Thalen, M.D., Chairman, Southeastern Ohio Committee on Trauma, was compelled to report: "The major drawback in handling this disaster was communications. The telephone system proved inadequate for assembling help and, if such a disaster were to occur when radio and television were not available, serious problems would result.

"As Holzer Hospital had no communication with the disaster area, it was handicapped in evaluating the situation and preparing for further casualties. Phones at the hospital were unreliable so that it was unable to communicate with the local radio station, firemen, and police. This situation needs immediate rectification."

Forty-six people died in the Silver Bridge disaster. It is not possible to say how many would have been saved if communications had not broken down. It is true, however, that the communication system did break down and 46 people died.

Communications and control soon became central considerations in the evolution of the Integrated Emergency Plan of the Province of Ontario Emergency Service Branch. Among the first moves was contact with the Provincial Department of Transport in order to secure the clear radio frequency necessary to tie all operations into a mutually supporting system. Ontario officials feel such a system must assure that a person needing assistance be aware of the means of gaining access to the control and dispatch systems. Intercommunication between base and ambulance crew, between ambulance crews and receiving treatment facilities, and during movement of a patient between the ambulance crew and other control centres *en route*. If the emergency unit in one hospital is overloaded, the dispatcher re-directs the ambulance to another hospital. Or, once the nature of the patient's condition is determined, an alert dispatcher can direct the ambulance to the best possible treatment centre. Valuable time is saved. The Ontario system also links all dispatching centres with hospitals as well as with police, fire departments, and The Emergency Measures Organization.

Emergency dialing systems also must be considered in any overall emergency communications plan. In North America, there have been many experiments with emergency dialing systems. Unfortunately, a two-year-old drive to introduce "911" as a United States nationwide telephone number for emergencies is running into unbelievable opposition. Only sixty-seven cities, nearly all of them small, have adopted the short number to make it easier for citizens to report emergencies. The system has won high praise in communities the size of Bountiful, Utah (population 6,000) and Yazoo City, Miss. (population 9,700). New York City is a major exception, but in most larger cities "911" has encountered wide official disfavour. In January 1967, only after prodding by the United States federal government, the American Telephone and Telegraph Company announced that "911" had been set aside as an emergency number and started converting pay phones so that no dime would be required for dialing it. But the system touched off strong resistance in police and fire departments. They insist on talking directly to any caller who has an emergency message for them.

It is not inconceivable that ambulances and emergency units will, in the future, be equipped with two-way television sets, permitting doctors attending emergency units and awaiting patients in transit, to monitor the patient and instruct paramedical aides at the scene of an accident or in the ambulance. Further, centralized computer banks containing medical case histories, similar to the progressive Swedish system, should be employed. Immediately upon identification of a seriously injured or ill patient, his history could be transmitted to emergency personnel treating the case.

Today, however, the fact is we have not yet admitted that well-organized communications are essential to modern emergency care operations.

On April 26, 1970, the Department of Transport in Washington announced the development of a basic training programme for ambulance personnel. Under provisions of the *Highway Safety Act* of 1966, the Safety Bureau developed and the Secretary of Transportation issued Highway Safety Program Standard No. 11 – Emergency Medical Services. The Standard requires states to establish criteria for types and numbers of emergency vehicles, including supplies and equipment to be carried and to set training standards for emergency personnel.

To assist the states in implementing the Standard, the Bureau is now providing guidelines of instruction for ambulance personnel. A survey conducted by various states estimates that such personnel currently numbers about 160,000 approximately 50 per cent of whom have had less than advanced Red Cross first-aid training.

In November, 1969, the Federal Government published the Task Force report, *The Delivery of Medical Care In Canada*. Much attention was paid to the deplorable state of community emergency response systems both in urban and rural areas. The report made a series of recommendations and outlined basic problems: "Far too often, in different regions, the response authority is sometimes hard or even impossible to identify in order to ensure co-ordination, assessment and supervision of the total emergency medical care program." "Too many physicians are not living up to their responsibilities for arranging for telephone calls during their absence or non-availability." The Task Force report provided some discouraging insights into the emergency care situation in Canada.

Let's face up to the problem and ask what real hope we do have that the present state of North American emergency care is going to improve in the relatively near future.

While we have seen some recent improvements at the community level, we have also seen that Washington has issued standards for emergency care which will require state co-operation. The federal department that issued these standards, the Department of Transport, is the same that issued standards for the building of safe cars. By dragging their feet and lobbying, the motor vehicle and allied industries have been so successful in watering down the standards that they are next to meaningless when compared with what could have been done. In the emergency care field, the Department of Transport issued *Emergency Medical Services Standards* in 1966. That was over five years ago, and we have seen next to no real progress. The issuing of federal standards often causes a momentary flurry of favourable newspaper and media comment. An unwary public mistakes this for concrete action – and an important battle in the war is already won by special interest groups. What was true with Washington's Federal Safety Standards for Motor Vehicles is now true with Federal Standards for Emergency Health Care Services.

The Task Force report recently published by Ottawa is a relatively extensive document and makes recommendations and proposals which are of high priority and could be initiated in the short term. Yet a closer look gives reason for skepticism. In typical fashion, the report largely calls for more research, more studies, and lots of co-operation between levels of government. As a result, the recommendations have a meaningless generality about them when it comes to action on specifics.

In the emergency health care field in both Canada and the United States, we need action on the community or regional level. If there is to be action, it will require great co-operation between an aroused public, active legislators, and a responsible medical profession. It will involve strong central policies which are flexible enough to account for particular local needs and local self-initiative. When it comes to real emergencies, we have long since learned that we cannot wait for Washington or Ottawa to act at the local level.

In the meantime, we can only wonder how and why a people who inhabit a continent such as ours, and who continually boast of North American technology, organization, and management techniques, can tolerate the state of our emergency services. Only the future will tell whether or not the medical profession working together with progressive legislators and an aroused public concern will bring about order and progress in a field which, after all, is a matter of life and death. Our life. Our death.

4
Discipline and Control

The medical profession has been granted the right to regulate itself, and while the majority of doctors are hardworking, honest, and truly dedicated, they are also fearful of competition, protective of an archaic system, and resist most innovations.
CENTRE FOR THE STUDY OF RESPONSIVE LAW

In community after community all over North America, medical tragedies have occurred which are remembered and still talked about by local citizens. As I grew up in Montreal a distinguished-looking gentleman named Thomas Stewart was often seen walking on the street. He was completely blind. As a young law student at McGill he experienced severe trouble with one eye. Subsequent diagnosis determined that the eye should be removed and Tom Stewart was prepared for surgery. Somewhere along the line, something went wrong. Stewart woke up in total darkness, a total darkness that was to stay with him for the rest of his days. The operating surgeon had removed the good eye.

A reasonable hope is that things have improved over the years and that modern surveillance procedures would not permit a repetition of the Stewart incident. Yet, it would be folly to be complacent.

One Life – One Physician, an inquiry into the medical profession's performance in self-regulation, was reported and made public by the Center for the Study of Responsive Law in Washington in the fall of 1970.

The report pointed out that the medical profession is a "unique and privileged one." In its hands lie the lives and well-being of all North Americans. The medical profession has been granted the right to regulate itself and while the majority of doctors are hard-working, honest and truly dedicated, they are also "fearful of competition, protective of an archaic system and resist most innovations."

Doctors are human and subject to error and within the profession there is a huge variance of individual competence – which means North American medical and health treatment runs from the superb to the downright dangerous.

24

Far too much of our North American performance is well below the best care available and few steps have been taken to guarantee minimum standards.

The very character of a profession militates against discipline or the regulation of its members. On the other hand, much of North American law prescribes many things the doctor may and may not do. He must use great care in prescribing narcotic drugs. He must report all still-births. He must notify the coroner of deaths occurring in suspicious circumstances. Yet, there is usually no routine policy for the policing and disciplining of the profession. In Ontario, for example, the College of Physicians and Surgeons relies exclusively on complaints, public reports and the professional grapevine.

Ontario's Supervising Coroner, Dr. H. B. Cotnam, has often complained about the province's inadequately staffed forensic medicine facilities. Not enough coroner's inquests are being held in cases where medical negligence is suspected. In one Ontario case, tissue slides which showed a woman of forty-six had died of strychnine poisoning were not examined by toxicologists until three or four months after her death. Cotnam has the opinion, by no means shared by all doctors, that an inquest should be held in all anaesthetic deaths. Under Ontario law, malpractice which necessitates an inquest is defined as failure of a professional person to render proper service through ignorance or negligence or criminal intent, especially when injury or loss follows.

Licence for the practice of medicine originated in the Middle Ages when the guild system provided a mechanism by establishing entrance standards for surgeons. Subsequently, medical faculties in the colleges and universities became the licensing authority for doctors. Medicine went through a laissez-faire period in the United States between 1820 and 1870 as most states repealed licensing requirements. Then quacks and low-standard medical schools were the order of the day. But after the Civil War, most of the states established boards of medical examiners. Currently, medical licensing is a "state right."

In Canada, licence to practice medicine is granted by the provincial authorities on their own terms, and there are significant variations from province to province. In Canada and the United States, varying degrees of discrimination from province to province, and from state to state, relating to place of origin, are at the basis of different licensing procedures involving foreign-trained students.

The section on Restrictive Practices in the Full Report of the

Committee of the Healing Arts (Province of Ontario), which was published in 1970, the Committee on the Healing Arts states: "Specific examples of protectionism as restrictive practices abound. The history of the professions discloses a general tendency which is unmistakable. In the admission to the profession, for example, we find a traditional general adoption of criteria for membership that are irrelevant. Discrimination on the ground of race, creed, place of origin has not been unknown." In fact, it varies from jurisdiction to jurisdiction. All licensing authorities in both countries have two major functions and responsibilities: the licensing of persons to practice medicine and the discipline of members already licensed.

Once the provincial and state bodies, at all times controlled by the medical profession, have authorized an individual licence, next to nothing is done to make sure the individual practitioner is working up to minimum standards. When he does damage, it's too late.

The Centre for the Study of Responsive Law's report asked some basic questions: What steps has the profession taken to evaluate state licensing, to oversee professional activity, and to ensure that those licensed remain fit to practice? The findings indicated gross inadequacies on the part of the profession to police itself. Take the case of continuing education of doctors and health personnel. With constant change and development in the art of medicine, its importance is obvious but neither the medical establishment, medical schools, or hospital authorities have taken any significant part in the continuing education of health personnel and doctors.

In 1961, the Medical Disciplining Committee, appointed by the Board of Trustees of the American Medical Association, reported its findings on the state of medical discipline and concluded that medical efforts largely cease with the discharge of the licensing function. Far too seldom are licensed physicians called to task by boards or societies. It has been estimated that 3 per cent of doctors present discipline problems, but that the figure would be substantially greater if one included those who do not live up to wider ethical standards.

The *New York Times* reported the account of the notorious Dr. Ronald E. Clark of Michigan. Before he was finally convicted of manslaughter in 1968, Clark had successfully avoided attempts to revoke his license. As early as 1956, the Michigan Board of Registration in Medicine acted to revoke his license. Over the course of many years, charges against him varied from moral turpitude, practising without a licence, to unprofessional and dishonest conduct, and finally

26

the charge that patients died unnecessarily under his care was brought against him. The case moved back and forth between courts and boards for years but Clark continued to practice medicine in Michigan. During this time neither the medical practice act of Michigan nor the courts protected the victims.

In many parts of North America, if a physician loses his hospital privileges, he can always work in a private office, a non-accredited hospital, or even start a hospital of his own.

The words "infamous conduct" still appear in the medical acts of several Canadian provinces. This is the case in Ontario and so only the most serious cases are tried. The nebulous wording of medical acts in both countries is widespread, and include such phrases as "unprofessional conduct," "conduct unbecoming a physician," "fraud and deceit in the practice of medicine." Obvious infractions, because of vague terms and language, go unpunished.

Licensing boards in Canada and the United States lack funds, staff and legal sanctions. Some boards have no investigating staff at all. In 1969, thirteen states, including Pennsylvania, reported no disciplinary action whatsoever by state boards. Even when boards do act, their actions are often meaningless.

There's a fascinating book called *Organized Medicine In Ontario*, a study prepared by Professor J. W. Grove of the Department of Political Studies at Queen's University, Kingston. In it is a listing of disciplinary cases heard by the Ontario College of Physicians and Surgeons over a five-year period. These included: a doctor who charged $20 for a death certificate; a doctor charged with misleading a patient by promising he could cure her of cancer; several doctors charged with fraud against a medical insurance plan; and several doctors charged with improper relationships with married women. The penalties ranged from suspensions, to reprimands, to being struck off the register.

Leaving the disciplining of doctors to an informal and indifferently organized mechanism established by the profession itself, and which rarely makes provision for consumer representation, is a denial of fundamental justice.

When referring to the standards of the profession, the code of the Canadian Medical Association is worth looking at. It is a curious mixture of highly general admonitions that could hardly be enforced, such as "the first consideration of the physician is the welfare of the sick." Some parts of the code seem not to relate to ethical matters at all. There are similar oddities in the International Code of Medical Ethics of the World Medical Association, a document bearing the strong influence of the American Medical Association. It describes as unethical "taking part in any plan of medical care in which the doctor does not have professional independence." The Canadian Medical Association code continually reflects an overwhelming concern for self-protection. It is inherent in the entire disciplinary apparatus.

The American Medical Association had a membership of 219,570 doctors as of December, 1969, out of a United States total of 325,000. Yet, it plays no real role and is not organized for ensuring the quality of the work performed by its members. Local grievance committees go into action only after the damage has been done. In 1969, forty-nine states (Oregon did not report) and D.C. had a total of only 161 disciplinary procedures. If a physician has been expelled from a state or county medical society, this does not prevent him from practicing, and the American Medical Association, or any other organization, does not have a central office to which all medical society actions are reported.

One recent study carried out in the United States determined that during physical examinations, 45 per cent of the doctors involved allowed patients to remain fully or almost fully dressed during the checkup. Seventy-four per cent performed no examination of the eyes, or only examined the surfaces.

It is most difficult to survey the quality of medicine practiced in the individual doctor's office. Invariably, the deplorable state of his records does not lend itself to proper surveillance. Frequently, the patient's charts and records remain the best clue to the quality of care received but frequently they are non-existent. Private practitioners' records in North America are usually inexcusably insufficient. Less than 20 per cent of these doctors keep what could be considered useful and meaningful records.

In 1912, Dr. R. C. Cabot of the American Medical Association presented a paper entitled "Diagnostic Pitfalls Identified During a Study of 3,000 Autopsies." He compared the post-mortem findings with the diagnosis and treatment found on the patients' charts and compiled tables which revealed scores of common diagnostic errors at the Massachusetts General Hospital. He required records to reveal these facts, yet today North American medical records are in virtual disarray. Even New York's Mount Sinai Hospital lost federal accreditation because its medical records were not in good order. The failure to keep records means no statistics for the establishment of basic, minimum standards.

Strict record-keeping can, and has, resulted indirectly from legal action. In a recent Quebec case it was found that a nurse had noted many warning symptoms but all she wrote down was "good enough day." That evening, the patient died. In the absence of adequate records, the court did not accept proof offered by the nurse, and the hospital was held responsible.

Prescription of non-acceptable drugs is another case in point. Excessive prescribing and types of drugs used are significant indexes of the quality of medical care. One United States study pointed out that at least 37 per cent of prescriptions examined were found to be non-acceptable, showing a further weakness on the part played by proper peer review in North American medicine. This is simply the regular or periodic review of a number of physicians' cases by other physicians, sometimes called medical auditing. Theoretically an excellent idea, today only lip service is paid to peer review as most physicians regard it as a punitive measure and don't like spying on each other, especially when they depend on other doctors for referrals.

In awarding $35,736 damages in a 1970 Quebec case where a little girl baby, Johanne Collin, was badly burned by a fluoroscope treatment, Judge Paul-Emile Roy said, "It would be surprising, to say the least, if the defendant could have followed this practice without certain of his colleagues in the same region or the same town becoming aware of it. If this was the case, it is unfortunate that they did not alert the College of Physicians and Surgeons."

A 1946 study entitled "Hysterectomy – Therapeutic Necessity or Surgical Racket?" examined two hundred and forty-six hysterectomies performed in ten hospitals, large and small, in three different states. The pre-operative clinical diagnosis of each patient was compared to the post-operative lab findings and the results showed 31 per cent of all women operated upon had no disease of the organs which were removed. Recently one young Quebec doctor told me he was assisting at surgery. The operating surgeon, getting ready to perform a hysterectomy, began his initial probing. There was a long, tense silence which soon turned to stark embarrassment. A hysterectomy operation had already been performed on the patient.

Wilfred English of Fort Erie, Ontario, died on November 22, 1970. During the autopsy it was discovered that a surgical towel measuring 30 inches by 18 inches had been left inside him after the operation. Subsequently, it was revealed that no count was taken of large towels before or after the operation.

In most hospitals, peer review simply does not take place effectively. Theoretically, it should involve the specific pre-operative consultation for each kind of operation, pre-operative visit and examination by the operating surgeon, and post-operative followup by the operating surgeon. It rarely does. The supervision of quality care by medical advisory committees leaves much to be desired. Medical audits and tissue committees are seriously affected by the pressure of work, staff shortages, and poor record-keeping.

5
The Doctorless Village

The doctors say that if they'd seen him sooner, Layton Coté wouldn't have died. . . .

No, I don't expect most of you to know the name of Layton Coté. But you might learn a lesson from his death. Layton Coté died a young man in December, 1969, and many people wondered why.

"He was here in the garage on Friday night around 8 o'clock and we were talking." recalls Charlie Labranche at his Esso Service Station in South Bolton, Quebec. "Layton," I said, "you'd better take care of yourself. Your eyes are looking bad!" "Yes," he said, "I think I'm coming down with the grippe. I'll go home, wash up, and go to bed."

The following Wednesday we buried Layton Coté.

According to Charlie Labranche, Layton Coté died of pneumonia. Others in the village say it was the flu, and the doctors say it was a brain hemorrhage that took his life. The doctors also say that if they'd seen him sooner, Layton Coté might not have died in his thirty-fourth year. That is very likely true but, you see, South Bolton doesn't have a doctor.

Once, Canada and the United States seemed full of small-town or country doctors. They were kindly, self-sacrificing men patiently making house calls, sitting at the bedside listening to a heartbeat through the stethoscope while the family anxiously crowded the bedroom doorway. No longer, however, is this the case.

South Bolton, where Layton Coté died, is one of many tiny communities nestled among the rolling hills of Quebec's Eastern Townships. Its people relied on the doctor from nearby Mansonville, until four years ago when Dr. Henry Gillanders died and no new doctor came to town to replace him. Today, when a person is sick at Mansonville and requires a doctor, it means a trip to Knowlton, seventeen miles away, where Dr. Richard Pellerin and Dr. Arthur Douglass have their offices, or across the border to North Troy, Vermont, where Dr. Leo Segal practices.

I know these details because they tell the story in my own area, but statistics show the same pattern exists across Canada and the United States and most country and small-town people are only too painfully aware of "Mansonvilles" in their own vicinity. From coast to coast, the doctor is disappearing from our villages and towns. Rural counties with populations of over twenty thousand, fifteen years ago, had five or six full-time doctors, now they have two and sometimes only one part-time doctor and soon they will have no doctor at all.

Much of the difficulty United States and Canadian small towns are having in replacing their family doctors stems from the fact that this kind of physician is a vanishing breed. Once, not all that long ago, the family doctor was an institution. As Frank Lowe, editor of Canada's *Weekend Magazine*, expressed it, "He delivered us, stitched us up when we got our face in the way of a speeding hockey puck, supplied us with some practical sex education and in certain instances made sure that a fellow could have a shot of booze (for medicinal purposes only, of course) when the government was doing its damndest to turn us all into teetotalers. Generally speaking, the family doctor was a bit of a character, an outspoken person."

On many occasions, the country doctor faced the sort of challenge only a Canadian climate could produce. For example, Mansonville's Dr. Gillanders often had to rely on a team of horses to make his calls. As the village grocer, Georges Hamelin, recalls, "Gillanders would hitch up his horses, sometimes at three o'clock in the morning, and head out over four feet of snow, and he knew he'd never be paid for it."

Another man cut from this same cloth was Dr. George V. Mc-Donald, who for years practiced medicine at the tiny crossroads community of Apple Hill which lies north of Cornwall in eastern Ontario. Dr. McDonald often made wintertime calls on snowshoes.

In a way, "Actor George" as he was known to everyone in the vicinity, was a perfect example of his breed. He was born in Apple Hill. When he had finished studying medicine in the city, he went back home and practiced his profession there for over forty years.

The medical practices of such doctors generally were administered in a rough-hewn way. It was like having an uncle who owned the local hardware store. When you needed something, you could go and get it, and generally he'd charge what he needed to make ends meet, and if you didn't get around to paying the account for a few weeks or months, well, the world didn't come to an end. "Dr. McDonald never sent out a bill to anyone," says Jean Guindon, owner of a cheese factory at Apple Hill, "and he never even marked it down. He just charged according to people's ability to pay, and according to his own needs, which were very modest."

"He was one of us," explained Guindon, "and when Doctor George died of a heart attack in July of 1969, everyone turned out for the funeral." Since that sad day, the community has been without a doctor. No one has come to take his place.

Because Canada and the United States face a general shortage of doctors, smaller centres are the first to feel the pinch as they can't compete with big city attractions in drawing medical men.

Trying to stem this tide, the community of Apple Hill, after several months without a doctor, banded together to form a citizens' Get-A-Doctor committee. Like countless other North American villages in the same predicament, there *is* medical help in the area, but not close enough to satisfy people who have grown up with the tradition of having a doctor on hand when an emergency arose.

For citizens of Apple Hill, today, the two nearest towns with practicing physicians are Maxville, ten miles to the north, and Alexandria, fifteen miles east. To get medical attention, a sick person has to be driven, or take a taxi. Says one resident of Apple Hill, "The kind of service we get is like when you have a sudden toothache and the dentist says he's busy but come along anyway and he'll try to fit you in between appointments." The inference, of course, is that between-appointment service is second-rate and examples of this are easy to find.

Another reason doctors are vanishing from our small towns is that these are the days of the specialist. But a village doesn't need an expert, it needs a general practitioner who can patch a cut, deliver a baby, or tend to the ailments of the elderly, as well as everything in between.

There are fewer and fewer general practitioners in the United States and Canada each year. To fill this gap, some medical schools are now starting a certification course in general practice, but this involves post-graduate training which takes three or four years and requires about as much time as a more lucrative, specialized field. So, all across the continent there are small towns and villages with no doctor at all.

As this reality strikes home, it grows clear that somewhere between unreasoning sentimentality. ("We always used to have our own doctor right here in the village, and that's how we still want it.") and ivory-tower efficiency, ("It's best to have these people come to the doctor, rather than vice-versa, since his time's too valuable and nowadays this is the most practical way to deliver health care,") there is a sensible compromise.

In Ontario, a compromise took the form of a government-sponsored programme, started in October, 1969, to provide a guaranteed annual income of $26,000 for physicians who would start a private practice in one of these communities. To qualify for this plan, a town must demonstrate to the provincial health department that it is a medically underserviced area.

Apple Hill happened to be the first village to qualify when the Get-A-Doctor committee prepared a petition with two thousand seven hundred names. Apart from the guaranteed annual income, Ontario provides grants of up to $14,000 to help establish practices, and partial payment of a medical student's fees. In return, the student practices for a year or two in underserviced areas after graduation. Even then, people in underserviced areas argue that while it is better than no service, why should they be singled out as the practicing ground for inexperienced doctors? As one young county general practitioner told me, "The word 'practice' is right. For the first years, I 'practiced' medicine in the truest sense of the word."

The Ontario Department of Health is now considering the feasibility of adding provisions to give these doctors free telephones, allowing municipalities to rent accommodation for them, and programmes for doctors to learn how to fly (as in the Flying Doctor Service in Australia). Yet, the whole incentive idea is far from being a success. After the programme had been operating for eight months, only 38 applications for contracts had been received and only eight were approved.

Apart from this "incentive programme," is there any other way enough G.P.'s can be found to make up the shortage in small communities? In most cases the answer is no, according to Dr. Don Rice, Executive Director of the College of Family Physicians of Canada. "We're engaged in trying to find more services for small areas," he says, "but we feel we're fighting a losing battle to get young people to go there. Young doctors are trained to work with other people and they tend to feel inadequate by themselves. Also, they want social and cultural facilities and good educational opportunities for their children which they simply can't find except in the cities."

34

What can be done about the problem? "We must make use of our improved transportation and communications" he says, "to develop new patterns of health care delivery." "For example," he suggests, "regional clinics could be set up to serve a fairly large surrounding area."

One doctor who has already done this is Raymond Robillard, President of the Quebec Federation of Medical Specialists, who runs a clinic in Sherbrooke, Quebec. In time, Dr. Robillard feels other clinics staffed by specialists could be located in many medium-sized communities, bringing a higher level of medical skill to rural residents than before. As it is now, when a critical case needs the attention of specialists, it invariably means difficult and time-consuming travel from outlying parts of a province or state to hospitals in centres like Montreal, Toronto, Winnipeg, Vancouver, Calgary and Halifax, New York, Los Angeles, Chicago or Boston.

There should also be smaller, more general clinics in communities of 3,500 to 5,000 run full-time by nurses and other paramedical assistants and visited by doctors on a regular basis. The vicinity around the clinic could be serviced by a public health nurse able to make house calls. In most cases she could take care of a patient on the spot, but she could also decide if he should see a doctor. Providing transportation to the clinics would be an important part of this approach. Ambulances, for example, would be needed. Obviously, a rural ambulance service would differ considerably from its counterpart in the city. It could be a regular, pre-arranged pickup service for important, but non-emergency visits to the clinic, planned to coincide with the doctor's visit there.

Operating with such clinics as their base, nurses could visit ailing elderly people, changing bandages, giving shots, in fact, performing almost all tasks now performed by doctors. Greater reliance on public health nurses and paramedical assistants in overcoming the doctor shortage is imperative in cutting down on valuable time wasted by those doctors we do have. But it requires a much more flexible attitude by the medical profession and it must come while the problem is still of manageable proportions.

"Doctorless villages" are not peculiar to rural areas. They can be found equally in the downtown core or poverty areas of our biggest cities. Within such neighbourhoods, often with a population many times larger than the towns which have attracted interest and attention due to their doctorless plight, are people desperately in need of medical care, but who find there is no doctor on hand to serve them.

This is part of the difficulty faced because of the extremely uneven geographical distribution of doctors. New York City, a "well doctored" area, had 278 doctors for each 100,000 residents in 1967. At the other end of the American scale, Mississippi had only 69. Even within the most favoured states, extreme distortions are common. Private physicians are as hard to find in some neighbourhoods of New York City as in the rural counties of the south. Over 412,000 people in 115 counties scattered through 23 states do not have access to a physician at all. In poor areas and ghettos in New York, only ten doctors care for each 100,000 residents.

Some may not wish to readily accept this concept of doctorless villages within our cities. Hospitals and doctors are easily reached by automobile, and the telephone is handy to seek transportation and help from police in emergencies, they argue. While this is undeniably true, the fact remains that many people in these areas don't succeed in breaking out of their villages for education, for employment, for cultural enrichment, or for health care.

Montreal's health department is fully aware of the appalling gap in health standards between those for our poor and those for the rest of the people.

Department officials know that low-income Montrealers die sooner than the rest of us, that many die quite needlessly, and that whole families live in physical misery that could be alleviated by more vigorous government action. They know, too, that unless the city's clinics and health services are expanded, perhaps hundreds of Montrealers will never live to see the 1976 Olympic summer games strictly because of official neglect. The Department's annual report usually skirts the more depressing comparisons of health standards between the poor and more prosperous areas of my city.

It has, however, never denied the separate findings of several social welfare organizations and university studies that have agreed on the present inequality of standards. What the Montreal City Health Department has *not* done is to take any practical steps to eradicate a deplorable situation which should bring shame to the city administration.

The University of Montreal has undertaken comprehensive health studies of the lower-income southwest sectors of St. Henri, Pointe St. Charles, and St. Jacques, a poverty ghetto of 120,000 persons. In St.

Jacques, for example, it found the death rate is one-and-a-half times higher and deaths from tuberculosis are thirty times greater than in the higher-income areas of the city.

In the entire area there are estimated to be only 28 full-time doctors serving 120,000 persons. That works out to one doctor per 4,500 residents, while the minimum requirements of the World Health Organization are one doctor per 600 population.

In New York City, where one is more accustomed to the idea of villages or ghettos, the experience of a Canadian-born doctor shows some dimensions of the problem. Doctor Harold B. Wise, now in his early thirties, was born in Hamilton, Ontario and graduated in medicine from the University of Toronto, moving to the United States in 1961 after a brief internship in Community Medicine in Saskatchewan. He was working at the Montefiore Hospital in New York, and soon grew so disgusted with the crowded conditions in hospital emergency rooms where the poor receive most of their treatment that he proposed a medical centre right in the very heart of the "doctorless village."

The idea received support from both his hospital and the federal government and Dr. Wise is now devoting his life to bringing medical care to 55,000 people in a depressing fifty-five block ghetto where poverty and its related ills are a way of life. He makes house calls to see patients, mainly black and Puerto Rican, who live among roaches, rats, and dogs in often dirty crowded and unheated apartments in the Bronx. They live in an area where lead poisoning and narcotic usage are of epidemic proportions, where until recently, the infant mortality rate was one in twenty-five and where tuberculosis and cancer have gone undiagnosed or untreated, or both.

Until Wise's Martin Luther King Medical Center was established in 1966, there were only three doctors to treat the thousands in this area. As a result, medical treatment, if any, was received in the crowded emergency room of a hospital some distance away. The centre now has twenty doctors and about four hundred employees, all recruited in the neighbourhood and trained there. They are handling what a recent report called an "onslaught" of three hundred patients a day, causing a fear that the centre will face increasing difficulty in fulfilling its twin objectives of medical care and preventive medicine.

When it was decided to open the medical centre, the first persons sent to the area were those who could teach local people the necessary skills, from nursing to taking X-Rays. It was eight months before a staff of sixty was ready and the doctors were sent in. Now the centre teaches a wide variety of subjects and claims that it can take a man with a Grade 4 reading ability and give him high-school training in six months.

One of its key functions is training "family health workers," persons trusted by the citizenry because they are from the area, who go to the homes and can uncover the causes of illness. At the same time these workers can give the doctors necessary background on patients and conditions in general. For instance, it is no use telling a patient to take medication three times a day after meals if it is known that the patient doesn't have three meals a day.

Lead poisoning from paint is another example. "All kids eat dirt off the floor. But if you do it in the Bronx you get lead poisoning and this causes brain damage, convulsions and death. We have an epidemic of lead poisoning in the Bronx," said Wise. The centre's health workers, who receive both legal and medical training, attempt to persuade landlords to re-paint apartments with a substitute for the cheap lead-based paint generally used.

Narcotic addiction is serious but he does not attempt cures, referring addicts to specialized agencies. It is a staggering problem, but Dr. Wise said that narcotics is only one problem of the ghetto where the citizens have a life span of nine years less than the average American. "Because their condition is undetected, more people die of cancer in the ghetto than elsewhere and the TB death rate is five times as high," he says. "The shocking part of it is that a lot of people are diagnosed but not treated." But Dr. Wise's courageous work has brought him hard-won rewards. He points with pride to the reduction in infant mortality since he started his practice. When he moved into the south Bronx, the death rate was 40 in 1,000. "Now because treatment is available," he said, "it is 3 per 1,000."

Back at centre-stage again, we come face to face with a key element in this whole dilemma of urban and rural doctorless villages. The doctor himself.

In rural areas, we know the general practitioner is vanishing. Many of the younger doctors are specializing in order to develop expertise in financially rewarding branches of medicine, as well as for the pragmatic reason of keeping up with their subject. A doctor from Sault Ste. Marie admitted to me that doctors also prefer to specialize, since this approach is more conducive to regular office hours, thus allowing a more peaceful and better-regulated life than the general practitioner falls heir to.

What about the plight of our doctorless rural areas? Dr. Richard S. Wilbur, Assistant Executive Vice-President of the American Medical Association, said, "The rural general practitioner in many areas is unsupportable and we shouldn't even try." Having said that, he apparently hadn't thought of any serious solution to the tragedy facing rural people. Rural people still feel there is much to be said for the family doctor, the family physician who can maintain the individual doctor to patient relationship based on some knowledge of the total family environment and background. Obviously, it isn't a bad concept but certainly it is only possible if we recognize certain realities. The fact is we have thousands of trained but disillusioned nurses, many now outside the profession, who could, with specialized training, perform almost all the functions of the old family doctor. Organized medical bodies who continue to resist this type of realism perform a great disservice to our society.

In the meantime, all over North America there is and has been a mass exodus of doctors from the low-income areas. In most cases the slack is never taken up by clinics staffed by trained paramedical aides and regularly visited by doctors. Often the rural poor lack the mobility to travel to larger centres for treatment and the results are disgracefully inhuman.

In the cities, too, doctors think of themselves in human terms when confronted with the whole problem of doctorless urban villages. Men like Dr. Wise in New York who plunge into the ghetto challenge with their shirt sleeves rolled up are only admirable exceptions to the rule. Doctors are human, too. They like to live where it's pleasant, just like anybody else. They aren't apt to be found in the downtown core.

As of now, in Canada and the United States, we need at least nine hundred well-staffed regional community centre clinics in the poverty areas of our cities alone. There is no indication at all that public authorities have begun to see these needs if spending estimates are any indication of intention.

Governments knew of the trend away from poor areas years ago. They knew that the doctorless village constituted a pattern for the future. Many state and provincial authorities actively discouraged doctors from practicing alone in rural areas as the standard of their

39

work could not be surveyed by their peers, yet next to nothing has been done to replace the vanishing doctor with trained paramedical assistants and with properly staffed clinics. Governments have poured billions of dollars into Medicare and Medicaid programmes for free services. Supposedly these programmes were designed mostly to assist lower-income citizens. Instead, rural people and the urban poor, those who suffered most in the past from the lack of health and medical services, have been dealt another blow. Government, while voting billions to help citizens pay for these services, failed to play their part in assuring the services were there in the first place. The cruel lunacy of this approach is there for all to see in our doctorless villages.

6
The Medical Manpower Mess

Doctors! Doctors run the 'non-system.' – SIDNEY LEE,
HARVARD MEDICAL SCHOOL

North American medical and health care services are close to complete breakdown. And one of the main reasons for this disastrous
situation is the critical shortage of medical manpower in general and
of doctors, or those who can perform the role of the doctor, in
particular.

If there are to be enough doctors to meet society's needs, the
medical schools must produce them. Medical schools must also have
teachers. Contemporary teaching faculties rely largely on a properly
funded research establishment which, in turn, depends upon enlightened public policies. Even if we had more doctors, the rightful distribution of their services depends on more community and regional
clinics and the comprehensive training of paramedical personnel. But
without full co-operation from both public and private sectors producing more doctors, will not, on its own, begin to cope with the
serious present maldistribution of services. Without a rational organization and management of hospital facilities, little can be done to
alleviate the situation.

The shocking state of North American medical services can, in
part, be attributed to the failure of university medical centres to provide an adequate research and education framework to ready the
young physician for his role in society. Governments, too, at all
levels, have consistently turned a deaf ear to warnings and have refused to vote funds for programmes to alleviate medical manpower
shortages. Finally, the medical profession's antipathy to change has
led to a serious shortage of medical health-care manpower, and an
absolute confusion in the organization of the manpower we do have.
The result is that in spite of the leap forward taken by medical science
in the last fifteen years, the lifespan of the average North American
citizen has not lengthened. In some instances, it has decreased. This,
in spite of the increased billions of dollars that have been poured into
the "non-system."

In all fairness however, there have been some giant strides in
medicine. We are told – and it would appear to be true – that medi-

cine has advanced more since 1935 than it had in all the history of mankind up to 1935. One hundred years ago life expectancy in Canada was below 40 years; in 1965 the life expectancy for male Canadians was 68 years, and 74 years for females. Prior to 1917, loved as the old family village doctor may have been, when it came to actual therapeutic measures, he had very few in his bag or his brain. Since those days, medical science has indeed made enormous progress, but society is receiving minimal benefits from it because of misguided public policies, and the incredibly short-sighted, collective selfishness of the medical profession.

While many facets are involved in the failure of North American medical manpower, one fact is obvious. We are running out of doctors at an alarming rate. When asked what was wrong with United States' medicine, Dr. Sidney Lee of the Harvard Medical School replied crisply, "DOCTORS! Doctors run the 'non-system'." Canada and the United States have given the medical fraternity much more freedom to police themselves than in any other country in the world. Yet doctors have been woefully slow to realize that, for years, society has looked upon proper medical and health care as a right, not as a commodity to be bartered and sold on the free market.

In the thirties, doctors hung up their shingles, and some waited a long, long time for their first patient. Slowly they would build up a practice. An old family doctor told me he sat and waited for days in his office for his first patient to call. One afternoon the bell rang and with eager anticipation he went to the door. It was a young boy with his pet cat which had been struck by a car.

Today, the tedious process of building up a practice has become a thing of the past. With the new voracious public appetite and the desperate need for medical services, the young doctor's waiting room is filled before he even has had time to frame his degree. Yet the medical profession's approach has not changed. Their restrictive attitude, conditioned by the hard times of the thirties, is based on groundless fears of over-supply. The Canadian Medical Association, the American Medical Association, and North American medical schools are the prime perpetrators of this dog-in-the-manger policy. And governments, by voting meaninglessly small sums for medical school staff and building facilities, must also share part of the guilt. To add to all this, the doctors themselves still resist innovation. The combined result is that unless we radically change the system, we shall continue to be faced with a medical manpower shortage of epidemic proportion for as long into the future as can be seen.

Dr. Daniel Federman, a renowned authority on the continuing education of doctors, says doctors are well aware of the fact that limited manpower resources are seriously hampering the delivery of service and are doing almost nothing about it. This is all the more serious because without the individual and collective help of doctors nothing much can be done to improve the critical shortage of medical manpower. There is no evidence, however, that they have any intention of changing on their own volition.

Today in the United States, there are 313,000 active physicians which, in effect, means that since 1950 the number of physicians has grown about 25 per cent faster than the total population. There has, at the same time, been a 10 per cent decrease in the number of active physicians treating patients in relation to the total population. The explanation for this is accounted for by the fact that the number of general practitioners, internists and paediatricians has fallen by one-third. The present ratio is 50 doctors per 1,000 of population. In the thirties, when the majority of doctors were in patient care and 70 per cent were general practitioners, a ratio of 135 per 100,000 population was thought to be desirable.

In the United States, at present, medical schools are now graduating approximately 8,000 students each year – 1,000 per year more than in 1960. It takes so much time and public money in both Canada and the U.S. to train doctors that even if tomorrow the number of schools were doubled, we would only have between nine and ten thousand extra physicians seven or eight years from now. If the United States were to have the optimum number of doctors (around 600,000), additional government costs would amount to $1.2 billion per year till 1985. All in all, by 1975, there should be between 370,000 to 380,000 doctors in the United States, an 18 per cent rise over 1965. Nevertheless, in both the U.S. and Canada, the trend will continue away from primary medical and doctor care, thus further compounding present difficulties.

The numbers of primary-contact physicians, general practitioners, paediatricians, and internists in Canada, continue their downward trend in relation to all physicians. They declined from 67 per cent in 1955 to 53.8 per cent in 1968. In 1967 and 1968 doctor registrations from immigration exceeded doctors graduating from Canadian medical schools, 1,213 to 925 respectively. Today 25 per cent of all Canadian physicians are immigrants, but with a world shortage of doctors we cannot expect this influx of doctors to continue. Such countries as India, Turkey and Iran have already taken steps to block doctor emigration.

Medical schools in both Canada and the United States are to be criticized. It has been shown that a much larger percentage of students state a preference for general practice when they enter schools than do at the end of their college training. Obviously curricula and the general university atmosphere plays a large role in this change. Teaching staffs are composed almost entirely of specialists, an increasing number of whom are full-time without any experience in family practice. It is the trend to specialization, to date, which has drawn and still draws doctors into the hospital environment away from the community.

Findings by one Canadian investigating team determined that we must develop more general-practice doctors, and that one year general or primary-contact practice be a pre-requisite for specializing.

The team also determined that more interns should serve in ambulatory care facilities as part of their training. The report confirmed that an overly centralized system orientated toward the hospital, drawing nearly all the doctors within its orbit, is one of the reasons we see such an uneven and unjust distribution of services and care.

Doctors spend an alarmingly large amount of their time on paperwork, bills, ordering supplies and keeping books. Group practice could stop a lot of this wasted effort, while organizing regularized primary contact and specialized treatment for the citizens of the area to be served. The advantages of group practice are obvious but with a few notable exceptions, the profession has rejected the idea.

Manitoba is an exception to the general North American rule. Fifty per cent of its doctors practice in groups. The advantages of this method have long been apparent, and any observer can only wonder why the idea is not readily accepted by the rest of the continent.

Many of today's solo practitioners are continually overworked and exhausted and this can and does seriously effect the quality of care that is available. Contemporary doctors' individual dedication to an outmoded delivery system has taken an unreasonable toll on their own health not to mention the health of their patients.

A number of enlightened Winnipeg physicians feel the advantages of group practice far outweigh the disadvantages. They stress that increased patient loads brought on by Medicare, with its accompanying work pressure, may reveal that group medicine is the only answer. The main resistance by solo doctors seems to come from pure selfishness. Overhead costs in the group take about one-third of their gross, compared with approximately one-quarter for those practicing medicine by themselves. It can only be hoped that, as doctors in both countries are now the highest earning group on the tax rolls, they will rearrange their priorities. What the group members buy is peace of mind, time to read and keep up with developments in the medical field, time to enjoy leisure and family life. Doctors are human. As one doctor at a special Winnipeg conference on the subject organized by Dr. Paul Thorlakson put it, "I don't know how else but in group medicine you can do this job, unless you want to kill yourself by breaking down with your first heart attack around forty and be under the ground by the time you're fifty-five."

The group practitioner also has ready access to consultation, or outright referral of patients to the other members of the group, as their special skills are required. More often than not, the group practitioner has his own group's modern laboratory and X-Ray department at his fingertips. This results in more rapid return of test results, more efficient patient care. The extra expense the group member incurs, compared with his solo-practicing counterpart, goes into pay cheques for people who relieve him of accounting, record keeping, obtaining supplies, paying rent and utilities. The doctor is free to concentrate on medicine.

Dr. Thorlakson believes group practice can provide a valuable training ground for medical students. "I am convinced," he says "that the faculties of medicine could, in the future, utilize the facilities of private group practice to great advantage, to broaden students' knowledge of medical practice away from the hospital environment." "It is neither necessary nor desireable that all education for practicing physicians, all clinical investigation and all basic research be initiated and directed by a faculty of medicine . . . university affiliation should be governed by the needs of the medical faculty and not by the plans and ambitions of hospitals."

Yet the medical profession in Canada and the United States have refused to adjust to essential change. It does not seem to understand the fact that it is moving into a working partnership with government, the public, and other agencies. The resistance to change has not only skyrocketed medical costs but has hurt the distribution of care services by the incredibly old-fashioned use of already insufficient manpower resources. Thorlakson asks some pointed questions which have obvious and often severe implications: "Should any medical institution or clinic close its doors at 6 p.m. each day and remain closed over weekends and public holidays? Are state financed hospitals and clinics to be encouraged to take over the practice of medicine as a result of the default of private physicians?"

Health-care teams could be another answer to the manpower and doctor shortage. They involve the organization of doctors working with other trained paramedical aides. Yet again, there is little reason to be optimistic about the likelihood of this method being implemented, and the present doctor-nurse relationship affords little eencouragement for the idea of greater co-operation. Obviously, outside forces must be brought into play to change these attitudes. If the situation is left in the hands of the medical profession, large segments of North American society will be deprived of doctor care almost entirely because of the doctor's selfish attitude toward protecting his affluent situation in life.

Medical licensing laws in almost all areas of the continent are weighed against the use of paramedical aides. In Ontario, doctors in many areas opposed the concept of trained paramedical help, even for emergency services, and, in California, charges for practicing medicine without a license have been laid against a neurosurgeon's assistant who, under instruction, removed stitches from a patient's incision.

With the crisis of inadequate medical care upon us, can we now look to Washington or Ottawa for hope? The answer, based on initial impressions must be a firm "No." Dr. James A. Shannon, former Director of the National Institute of Health, and currently a professor at the Rockefeller University in New York City, cited medical education as an example of the "inadequacy" of current and projected federal health programmes:

> There seems to be no high level appreciation of the fact that the shortage is truly great and is likely to become much greater in the immediate future. More importantly, there seems to be a lack of general awareness that the simple and modest extension of the present programmes, even when coupled with new programmes aimed at the evolution of new careers (*i.e.*, physician assistants), will not resolve the combination of shortage and maldistribution in any reasonable period of time.

These programmes were started much too late and are much too small to have any significant effect in alleviating the shortage of physicians.

At the most, the United States' Department of Health, Education and Welfare medical school programmes in fiscal 1969 and 1970 will result in a combined total of 1,600 physicians in 1975 and 1976, an increase of slightly more than one-half of one per cent in the current physician population. Furthermore, Dr. Shannon pointed out, these new physicians are "likely" to distribute themselves within the society in much the same fashion as the present physician population. "It is difficult to see what this small annual increment can be expected to accomplish." New types of health professionals such as "clinical associates" or "physicians' assistants" have stirred considerable speculation. Yet they won't be ready for action, even in small numbers, until 1974. The 8,000 physicians and 50,000 nurses who graduate each year could help medically deprived areas, but only if there were specific control of their deployment. Tragically, this is not taking place.

The present deployment deficiencies have been repeatedly stressed by the managers of federal health programmes and some private groups since the late 1950's. One can only conclude that the present programmes are timid rather than bold, stereotype rather than innovative, and reflect a low national priority.

In considering North America's serious medical manpower shortage, whether we are talking about group practice, more clinics, the team approach, training paramedical help, or producing more general practitioners, neither the attitudes of public and private sectors, nor the continuing perpetuation of over-lapping and unco-ordinated programmes give much reason for any real hope. Moreover, in the medical and health-care field, the critical manpower shortage sadly effects those who can least afford to be affected. It is thus with deficiencies in other social and economic programmes. It is thus that our so-called democratic society and its institutions will be judged.

7
The Medical School

He who knows only medicine does not even know medicine.

Until the beginning of the nineteenth century, the role the hospital played in medical education on this continent was small. Doctors were trained by the apprentice system with an individual physician teaching an individual student. The nineteenth century saw the founding of medical schools by groups of practicing physicians, usually associated with either universities or hospitals. These proprietary schools of medicine grew rapidly and by the turn of the present century, more schools of medicine were in existence than the one hundred or so which operate today.

In the year 1909, the Carnegie Foundation organized a survey by Abraham Flexner. For two years he visited, unannounced, faculties of medicine in the United States and Canada, following which he wrote a scathing report on the quality of the educational process. His report contained three main points. First, most of the proprietary schools of medicine which were in operation should cease teaching immediately. Second, practically no schools on this continent were providing a satisfactory academic atmosphere for the teaching of physicians. Third, never again should the teaching in any department of a medical school be done by physicians who receive their remuneration from other sources. A full-time teaching staff in each department was necessary.

The report provided a tremendous incentive to making schools of medicine a part of universities, and also attaching themselves to hospitals, which could be used for practical teaching. Flexner's efforts produced general improvement, at least in the early years. By the mid-sixties, the overall scene had deteriorated once more, and in 1968 there was a call to action by United States deans of medical schools and faculty representatives. Their conclusions were varied and far-ranging. The following were among their main points. (1) Schools must increase their output of physicians by increasing the number of enrolled students. (2) The schools must also admit more students from those geographic areas, economic backgrounds and ethnic groups which, up until then, had been inadequately represented. (3) Education of the physician should be individualized, to fit the students' varying rates of achievement, educational backgrounds and career goals. (4) Curriculum should be developed by inter-departmental groups that include students. (5) They should be ratified by the faculty as a body, rather than by individual departments, thus minimizing repetition.

Flexner's report of 1910, and the American Association of Medical Colleges' report of 1968, both undertook the significant task of bringing medical education into a relevant relationship to the major changes which had already taken place in society. Early in the century, it had been necessary to bring the methods of biophysical science into medical practice by moulding medicine into a university discipline. Today it is necessary to bring behavioral, social and managerial expertise into medical education, as well as an understanding of health care, so that they may better serve the student, the patient and above all, the people.

Even in the future, the doctor or his replacement will continue to be the central or leading figure on "the team." The doctor's performance and attitudes will always keynote activities in medical and health care sectors. How he, or she, has been taught to think and act at the medical school level is of obvious and paramount importance.

While North American universities can claim much of the credit for the improvement of services, they most certainly share a great deal of the blame for the current crisis in medical manpower. They are not facing up to their dual role of preserving worthwhile traditions and bringing about innovation. Medical teaching is not being dovetailed with large mass movements in technical research and in social change. Many students and young doctors today are interested in helping the needy and underprivileged. They want to work, at least in part, as "storefront" doctors. They want to integrate medical care with practical efforts to improve the welfare of families and communities. But they are often thwarted by the dead hand of tradition that pushes them in the direction of competitive private practice. They rarely receive stimulating leadership in the university environment, which tends to remain aloof from social issues. Its officials, responding to criticism with an air of superiority or arrogance, are still copying eighteenth-century methods, whereby a physician who aspired to be a gentleman received a university degree, permitting him to practice as a scholar largely among the "upper classes."

The lecture, the laboratory exercise, and the clinical case method remain the *modus operandi* of medical teaching. Suggestions that the subject matter of medicine might be approached differently, or that it can include economics and the social sciences are met with parochial resistance. There are a few exceptions.

One is McGill University in Montreal, where the "New Man" concept for doctors was recently initiated. In co-operation with four American medical schools and heavily funded by American foundations, the McGill school began in July, 1970, an experiment with medical education designed to create a "new man," whose special talents and expertise are desperately needed at all levels of government, as well as by medicine itself.

With the graduation, in about three years, of the first three trainees, there will appear in Canada for the first time a doctor who is both fully trained as a physician and also competent in such areas of the social sciences as economics, political science, sociology, systems engineering, computer technology and business administration. Dr. John Beck, chairman of McGill's Department of Medicine, said that, until now, nobody has been trained to solve the border-crossing problems which exist between medicine and the social sciences, and which continue to perplex the growing ranks of those concerned with the health and welfare of citizens. Beck feels "the development of such men, who will be known while in training as clinical scholars, is crucial and the fact that virtually none have been trained means we are behind the times."

Curriculum is another serious question constantly under review. Dr. J. Wendell MacLeod, Executive Director of the Canadian Association of Medical Colleges, feels "the curriculum too often tends to be looked on in its most physical sense, a timetable of hours, subjects, and departments, rather than as the expression of a certain amount of past as well as present educational philosophy and the reflection of a great many circumstances both within and without medicine."

When seen as a matter of content, the question of curriculum looks like a race no man can win, and the information explosion has made traditional methods obsolete.

From 103 responses to a questionnaire sent to 117 United States and Canadian medical schools in 1967 and 1968, it was learned that practically all had made some curriculum change, or planned to do so. A key trend was to individualize the student's learning experience. Two-thirds of the reporting schools defined a minimum "core" of compulsory learning experience, leaving more time for other subjects.

Most investigations have shown medical school faculties to be intolerably departmentalized, and specialized, causing unnecessary overlapping and duplication in courses. Recommendations from these inquiries, without exception, point to the fact that all curriculum should be controlled by general faculty.

In the learning experience for students, there is far too much rote and repetition, while in the lab they follow what one student called "cookbook instructions." The result is passivity, as the professor dispenses knowledge, and the sponge-like student absorbs it and squeezes it out on command. At the same time, increasing specialization in scholarship has made for the fragmentation of knowledge and narrowing of the overall view. The scientist finds himself in increasing isolation, separated not only from other branches of learning, but even from other specialists in his own general field. Watching cardio-pulmonary physiologists and basic endocrinologists trying to understand one another illustrates the point only too well. As a result, the medical school has been dubbed by many as a federation of autonomous departments, in which students suffer from duplication and disharmony of teaching.

The objective of any field of professional education is to equip future practitioners with both science and art, that is, both knowledge and skill. During those times that knowledge and skill have been developing somewhat independently and at essentially similar rates, it has been possible to separate the preparation into two categories, education and training. As an example, the preparation of the future physician has been divided into pre-clinical years and clinical years at the undergraduate level; internship and residency in the graduate experience; and finally, the post-graduate education of the practicing physician. This convenient and sharp fragmentation is no longer possible. Knowledge and skill have begun to interact without a time lag.

The arbitrary division of medical education into pre-clinical and clinical experiences is still too prevalent in many North American medical schools. The two are inseparable in practice and, as such, should be taught that way, not in isolated correlation seminars, but in fully integrated lecture series and laboratory experimentation and demonstration, beginning in the first year of admission to the college of medicine. It is hard to understand the logic behind a programme that provides an immense volume of material that must often be subject to rote learning for exam purposes, and yet makes no provision for repeated assessment of the student's ability to apply this material to the problems with which he is ultimately to deal.

Some students find the current transition from pre-clinical to practical clinical work inordinately difficult, a typical comment being, "I came to medical school to be a doctor, but I didn't see a patient until two years later." Students have their enthusiasm dampened by being kept away from practical problems, and many have become dissatisfied and frustrated with the irrelevance, duplication and lack of flexibility in their studies; the lack of human contact and social concern in their educational experience; and with their isolation until their fourth year from the service aspects of medicine. Much of their anger is directed at university educators. They feel the university is an ivory tower, not only isolated from society, but from medicine too.

People become sick, are cured, or die outside the school. Memory work and didactic lectures are probably the most wasteful, unrewarding and dehumanizing methods of education. Yet, they are the mainstays of rigid university curricula. The training of a whole generation of doctors has become increasingly inadequate and frustrating.

The scientific process has had a tendency to depersonalization in medical care. With fascinating new tools to study heart action and renal function it was easy to forget that the owner of those organs was a person, who was important not only to himself but to a family and a community as well. Medical education has become increasingly hospital-centred with attention focused on major illness, on the problem case, and on highly technical investigation. The student has been encouraged to think of health care in terms of dealing with acute illness, rather than as a continuing and responsible concern for the maintenance of health by watchful prevention. Medical students all over North America realize that in the early seventies, new patterns of interaction between people, students, and teachers are a crying need. For five years now, the student health organizations in United States' and Canadian medical schools have moved ahead of most faculties, coming to terms with low-income areas. Student health organizations, students in medical nursing, social work and education, are spending their summers in health care and community development projects, which they have organized in co-operation with social agencies, parish clerics and nearby doctors.

The McGill Student Health Organization opened a storefront medical clinic in July, 1968, in Montreal's inner city. Students of medicine, nursing and sociology, along with volunteer physicians from three teaching hospitals, gave personal care to a largely poor population. In British Columbia, students in medicine and nursing have played the role of "health ombudsman" while working with the inner city service project in Vancouver. The 1969 Appalachian Student Health project (s.a.m.a.) in many ways typifies current medical school student activities. The Appalachian Project was developed by the Student American Medical Association in an effort to create a sustained programme which would provide an educational experience in rural medicine. It was also hoped that these experiences would convince the student of the desirability of practicing rural medicine – preferably in Appalachia. s.a.m.a.'s further intention was to make the students fully aware of the inadequacies in their medical curricula, which limited their exposure and learning experiences in the whole area of health care for the poor, both rural and urban. The hope was that they might be able to influence medical school and nursing curricula to provide more people interested in, and appropriately trained for, the health needs of rural America.

While the North American medical school scene is an easy one to find fault with, all the blame should not be directed to the schools themselves. For some time, North American medical schools have been asked to plan their future growth without knowing how much money they could spend. For example, no Canadian medical school directors know how much money will be available from Ottawa for the period 1970-1975. This means there is no real basis for decisions or for future planning.

The federal government's Health Resources Fund was created in 1966 to help provide money to meet capital costs of constructing, renovating, acquiring and equipping health training and research facilities. Five hundred million dollars were made available for use over a fifteen-year period. The fund was to pay up to 50 per cent of costs, with the rest provided by the provinces or some other source. In December, 1967, things got off to a bad start. Finance Minister Sharpe announced at that time that he would seek to limit the total fund allocation in the next fiscal year to forty million dollars. In fact, the total actually approved was $37.5 million. The same limitation was applied for the 1969-1970 fiscal year. This mid-stream change in rules has created chaos with the programme. In the fund's first nine months, from July 11, 1966 to March 31, 1967, federal and provincial health officials agreed that $14.9 million should be given to various projects, but only $4.7 million was actually paid out by March 31, 1967. In the following fiscal year, another $66.3 million was committed, and payment only totalled $32.6 million.

In Canada, at least, central to the operation of most provincial Medicare plans was the regionalization of medical and health services. The Province of Quebec, for instance, under the terms of the Castonguay commission for medical and health services, has been divided into three regions centering around Montreal, Quebec, and Sherbrooke. Integral parts of such regionalization plans were, and are, health training centres, with university affiliation where doctors and most other paramedical workers would be trained. The fact that such centres were not in full operation, or even initiated, when the Quebec Medicare plan got underway means breakdown and complete dislocation of services in the immediate future.

Health science or training centres with university affiliation surely are a sign of future trends. Too often, the doctor has been trained in isolation, away from those paramedical workers with whom he must work and co-operate with after graduation. Too often, the paramedical worker has, likewise, been trained in isolation. Universities which have, as well as a faculty of medicine, faculties in other health science fields, will increasingly group these schools in "Health Science Centres." Universities should co-operate with the out-patient departments of teaching hospitals in teaching total health and medical care needs for the individual in a community setting. Year-round medical schools should be considered, and more students should be channelled into the area of primary physicians.

To provide such education, those charged with the responsibility for directing educational institutions, medical, nursing, and dental schools, universities, and the like, must participate jointly in planning for the whole of professional education. Each institution must understand its role and the relationship of that role to all of the other parts of the programme and strive to articulate that part to the whole.

It must now be obvious that medical schools can only fulfill their responsibilities to society with dramatic change. When medical education is devoted, not to prior conceived notions of the educational needs of the student, but to the health and medical care needs of the people, the advancement of humane understanding and the welfare of the community – then, and only then, will our society begin to produce useful practitioners of medicine.

8
North American Medical Research

They (medical scientists) go not because they want to leave Canada but because opportunities for study and research are better in the United States.

The story of Wilder Penfield and the Montreal Neurological Institute is now legendary. For three decades before his retirement in 1960, this world-renowned neuro-surgeon gave Canada and Canadians something to be proud of. Penfield, by the strength of his character, determination and foresight, built, on the slopes of Mount Royal overlooking the city of Montreal, a research team in neurosurgery and neurology second to none in the world. Students and scientists from all over the globe flocked to the Institute, which owed much of its support to prestigious American foundations, but toward the end of the fifties, it became apparent that such support, alone, was not sufficent for the orderly growth of this world-renowned research centre.

In the spring of 1959, Penfield forwarded to me, in my Ottawa office, a lengthy memorandum outlining some of the problems at the Institute. His main concern was the Institute's dependence on yearly short-term grants from the federal government, and he was finding it more and more difficult to build continuity into its research pro-grammes. He argued for a federal endowment policy of research assistance so that "stability and continuity" could be built into long-term projects. I made a summary of his recommendations and went over them with Prime Minister John Diefenbaker. A meeting was arranged and attended by Penfield, a few of his colleagues, the Prime Minister and some other cabinet ministers. The outcome was a major disappointment to Penfield. The government continued its broad sup-port of the Institute, but rejected any endowment policy on the grounds of its inability to earmark funds in perpetuity, and on the further grounds that it would be setting a precedent which might easily have to be applied to other research activities.

Both Ottawa's and Washington's on-again/off-again attitude to the funding of medical research has created the kind of uncertainty which has made it extremely difficult to build top-level excellence into a research team.

Canada has a long history in the field of medical research. The most notable of the medical pioneers was Michel Sarrazin, chief surgeon to the French troops at Quebec. In 1799 he was made a corresponding member of the Académie Royale des Sciences de France in recognition of his contribution in the field of botany, largely brought about because of the early dependance on natural drugs.

In the nineteenth century, post-graduate medical training for Canadian doctors generally meant travel to Europe or the United States. Only slowly did Canadian medical research labs build up. It was in this context that significant work was done by such pioneers as Osler, M. Abbott, A. B. MacCallum and A. T. Thomas, but Canada's achievements in medical research were, however, scarcely noticed at home or abroad until, in 1921, the isolation of insulin by Banting, Best, Collip, and Macleod at Toronto suddenly claimed the attention of the scientific world.

The dramatic research achievements in medicine during the Second World War created an atmosphere favourable to the expansion of medical research and in 1948, the federal Department of National Health and Welfare instituted a system of health grants, part of which was used to promote university research.

Today, the scene is far from encouraging. The blame lies in three directions – government rejection of responsibility, the research community's poor organization, and public apathy. Let us examine the situation.

If a country is to enjoy the full benefits of science, one fact is clear. It cannot afford to depend on the initiative of others. It must have its own research base and scientific effort. The arguments which suggest that Canada is too small to produce the personnel and technology necessary for first-rate medical research are both inaccurate and dangerous. We simply cannot import scientific discoveries, and the technology we require in the field of medicine, as we do in other industries. The facts are that we just could not recruit teachers for our medical schools if they were to be merely purveyors of knowledge, rather than contributors to knowledge. An even more important reason lies in the fact that we cannot "buy" all our medical science and technology because scientific knowledge can be imported and used profitably only by countries that themselves have a sufficiently large body of highly trained specialists. There are some notable exceptions, however. For example, a newly-developed vaccine may be imported and safely administered according to instructions. On the other hand,

56

the benefits of the artificial kidney cannot be made available in every hospital simply by distributing the necessary machines. The successful application of this form of treatment requires the presence of a specialized team, only to be found at present in those centres doing research in the field. Topflight surgeons are needed to apply techniques, immunologists to know when tissues are accepting or rejecting a transplant, and biochemists to know when to trust or distrust results. Without these people, the process can't be taught or applied.

As recently as 1966, authorities noted that Canada's standard of health care was dangerously close to slipping quickly and quietly to the level of "the second rate." In 1966, it was only too apparent that future Medicare schemes were about to usher in a new era of increased needs. At the same time, four of Canada's medical schools were in danger of losing their accreditation as unfit teaching institutions. A quarter of our newly graduated doctors were going to the United States each year.

As medical research goes in Canada, so goes the quality of our medical schools and the quality of our medical and health care. In 1966, Canada had approximately 1,200 teacher-scientists actively engaged in health research and in teaching new professional personnel. To meet the minimum requirements for new medical personnel in the 1970's, it was advocated that the number of teacher-scientists had to rise to at least 2,400 by 1970. Initially hopes were high and Ottawa and the federal authority made new promises for increased assistance to medical research. The dreams were shattered when the Treasury Board froze the annual assistance figure at a mere 20.5 million dollars. Then as now, the crucial factor in attracting and keeping topflight researchers and teachers was and is the provision of adequate facilities and research funds. Yet, for the brilliant young medical graduates who become the staff members needed by our medical schools, the lure of the United States is very strong. In one year, in the mid-sixties, 19 out of the top 20 of the medical graduates from the University of Manitoba went to the United States. That same year, 49 per cent of all Canadian medical graduates left for south of the border. Even now, 25 per cent of the 900 doctors graduating each year from Canadian medical schools leave for the United States.

They go, not because they want to leave Canada – most don't – but because opportunities for studies and research are greater in the United States. Frequently it's the best who go, because adequate financing provides a productive research environment in the States.

The United States spends about $6.50 per capita of public funds on medical research each year. Canada spends $1.05.

Somehow or other Ottawa refused to recognize that only first-class teacher-scientists will insure first-class doctors and that this is, at least, a large part of the formula for "excellence."

Dr. John Evans, * Dean of McMaster's new Medical College in Hamilton, Ontario, noted his troubles in the summer of 1966. "I need about ninety-five teaching-scientific staff for the school by 1969. I've contacted fifty to sixty potential recruits, mostly in the United States, without much luck. Canada is losing the battle to hold researchers. Very few top medical scientists stay in Canada today because of the scientific environment. If they stay, it is because of the social influences. I would say there are not more than ten pretty good medical-research teams in the country."

From 1946 to 1965, Canada produced 1,300 Ph.D.'s in the medical sciences. The United States grabbed up one-third of them, including most of the best. In the prevailing climate in Canada, adequate research support, reasonable security, expanding opportunity and the other attributes of a healthy scientific environment seems almost beyond hope.

Many Canadian-born scientists want to return to Canada, but only if the opportunity is there. As one U.S.-based Canadian scientist confirmed, "A person tends to look at the nature of the post rather than the country in which it is located." Medical research is now a team effort and our emigrants seek association with men of international reputation in an academic or scientific community that values the research-orientated individual. At present, Canada has opted for mediocrity.

What about a medical research science policy for Canada? The Canadian Special Senate Committee on Science Policy, which reported in the fall of 1970, clearly demonstrated that Canadian federal authorities had no general science policy with integration and direction, and absolutely no policy at all for scientific research in the medical field. The report made the following points: (1) Much of Canada's $1 billion annual expenditures on science is wasted or squandered. (2) There is a complete lack of coherent science policy. (3) Because of departmental rivalry and the veto power of the Treasury Board, the Federal Government has operated on the basis of a series of limited and isolated science policies with no overall view of what is going on and a global strategy for what has to be done. (4) Agencies in

* Dr. Evans has since become President of the University of Toronto.

many cases have lost sight of their original job and refused to cut programmes that have failed and hundreds of millions of public funds
have been wasted.

At least part of the blame for current problems facing the North
American medical research community must be placed at their own
doorstep. It is not peculiar to Canada or to the world medical science
establishment, but because of inadequate arrangements for co-ordination within the medical science community, major breakthroughs
take an inordinately long time to receive wide distribution.

Many critics have noted the appearance of a stifling bureaucracy
within the North American medical research establishment. In many
cases, in order to attain a certain rank and obtain grants from the
public purse, an individual researcher must have so many "bodies"
working under him. The implications are obvious.

Up until now, the medical science communities both in Canada
and the United States have devoted little or no attention to identify-
ing the problems or needs in the health science or research system,
with the needs of education and service to the community. Of course
in many cases it is our faulty delivery system which retards the passage of benefits to the population at large. According to Dr. Preston
Robb, Neurologists-in-Chief of the Montreal Neurological Institute,
many victims of epilepsy aren't benefiting from current knowledge
about the treatment and control of the disease. "Many epileptics," he
said, "are poorly treated because they're not getting the best of what
is available. We need better delivery of medical care for these people."

According to Robb, children with absence or *petit mal* attacks
are frequently treated with drugs which are effective only in cases of
major epilepsy. There are specific drugs for the treatment of *petit
mal*. The consequences are unforgivable.

The ultimate goal of health research, not discounting its pure
intellectual worth, should be to improve the medical and health care
of the community.

Science has flourished remarkably in the United States since the
Second World War largely because of the intelligent use of public
funds. Unfortunately, during this time, the science community did
little to communicate its goals to the public. The opportunity was
missed to capture public imagination and support. Based largely on the
work of then-Health Educator and Welfare Secretary, Marian Folsom, Congress gave uncritical support to biomedical research funding.

However, in the late fifties, attitudes to the project grant system of research support was affected unfavourably by the trend of popular interest and attention on specific achievements. In the field of cardio-vascular medicine, for instance, it has been more convenient to view research progress in terms of the progression from "blue baby" operations, through complex vascular surgery and open-heart surgery to, finally, heart transplantation than to consider the best scope of the inner-related basic scientific effort that necessarily preceded each of these achievements. It is simpler to raise funds for quite explicit programmes, which tend to be short-term, such as the testing of a specific drug, than for longer-range and more complex studies, that are more general in nature but are necessary if substantial advance is to be achieved.

As in Canada, just at a time when U.S. universities are beginning to define and understand their social responsibilities and to understand the relationship of medical research to these responsibilities, the Federal purse snapped shut. Recession and competing demands brought about by social turmoil in the cities, escalation in Vietnam war commitments, all were part of the cause, but it was not difficult to close the purse because public involvement in the programme had never been developed.

Beginning four years ago, in the U.S., the increases for support of research through the National Institute of Health became less than the cost of living increases.

The United States federal budget estimates for medical research funding are $38 million over the expenditures for fiscal 1970, but they are far below anticipated increases. This means many research projects are about to be abandoned and many expensively trained young medical scientists, ready to make significant contributions, will soon be without work.

Morale is at an all-time low in the United States and Canadian research establishments. In Canada, 6 per cent of the G.N.P. is devoted to the health services system, yet there is clearly no national science policy for health. Nobody, either within or outside government circles, seems capable of any attempt at all to articulate such a policy. Thus we have witnessed an unco-ordinated expansion of facilities, and excessively expensive arrangements for the delivery of health care.

Recent cutbacks in Canadian federal support for medical research have come at a time when the infrastructure of a broadly-based Canadian research effort has largely been pulled together and Canada was beginning to see a degree of excellence in its medical research build-up. Today, as more and more specific projects face termination, young scientists get ready to leave the labs.

As late as February, 1971, the world-famous scientist, Dr. Hans Selye of the University of Montreal spelled out the problem. He claimed recent decision to cut back could cause "irreparable damage" to the future of medical research in Quebec. Best-known for his work on the effects of stress, the director of the University's Institute of Experimental Medicine and Surgery said he could not replace the people who have left. The war in Vietnam, said Selye, had also directly affected the amount of medical research being carried out at his institute. Before the war, 80 per cent of the institute's budget was provided by the u.s. National Institute of Health and 20 per cent by Canadian sources. Because of the war, recent grants by the u.s. to Canada have been severely limited.

In periods of economic recession, government officials attempt across the board cutbacks on expenditures and programmes which are not permanently built into Federal budgetary expenditures. Some of the shameful research waste brought about by the indiscriminate pruning and cancelling of expensive projects only half underway or completed is hard to imagine. Moreover, they are pruned or cancelled, in the case of Canada, by Treasury Board officials who have no idea whatsoever of the ramifications or goals of individual medical research projects and their relationship to the total national health and medical picture.

Cancer kills 330,000 North Americans every year, yet between 1968 and 1970 cancer research funds in the u.s. were cut by 30 per cent.

Heart research projects are also being cut by the present administration. An example: For twenty years, more than five thousand people in the Boston suburb of Framingham have been willing subjects in a heart disease research project. The project has been remarkably successful, producing most of what is known about the causes and prevention of heart disease, North America's leading killer. But, as of July 1, 1970, the study budget was cut sharply in a controversial decision by the United States government.

In the twenty years that the Framingham Heart Study has been underway, a clearer portrait has gradually emerged of the now familiar candidate for a heart attack. He is a flabby, middle-aged male given to excesses – too much to eat, too much to drink, too many cigarettes, too little exercise, a tendency to diabetes. He may feel perfectly well but he may already have had a silent heart attack and be unaware of impending disaster.

When the project began in this small community, 5,127 men and women between thirty and sixty-two were enrolled, all volunteers. Since then, each has been given an extensive physical examination every two years. Now, however, the research staff is being reduced, eliminating the biennial physical examinations, undermining the research programme.

"Colossal blunder," said Dr. William B. Kanner, director of the heart study, "I think it's a tremendous waste of a potential national resource that could be exploited."

With the Framingham population moving into advanced years, Kanner said, there is an opportunity to learn not only more about heart disease and stroke, but such things as senile mental deterioration, emphysema, cataracts, and deafness.

To do this kind of research correctly, he said, the work should start early, before the onset of the illnesses, as with his Framingham group. "We have already their living habits and biology" he added. "We can see if there is any relation to intellectual function. What's different about the person who ends up mentally deteriorating? . . . We're not going to find any tincture of youth, but we have to find out how to keep people hale and hearty and vigorous up into old age, until they fall over dead. We should literally study this group to death."

Up until now, in North America, far too few of the fruits of the health sciences have been made available to citizens. In many cases nothing should be allowed to slow down the contemporary thrust of our research projects. Heart transplant research is a case in point. The paradox of our age is the enormous gap between our scientific knowledge and skills and our organizational arrangements to apply them to the needs of man. Medical research must begin to realize the importance of its relationship to and integration with education and service to the community. At the outset, this means setting up communications between the health sciences and with society as a whole. This won't be easy. More medical scientists and researchers are at work in the world now than the combined total of all the medical scientists in past history. The very volume and mass of research literature makes communication and co-ordination difficult.

The challenge of better communication to the public by the scientific community is still largely unmet, yet must be faced up to if biomedical research is to receive the necessary public support. When the goal is out of sight, the community soon forgets the importance of government support of medical research. The main weakness of the federal support system for biomedical research has been failure to integrate it, at least in the public mind, with education and service. Today the science community must make the public realize that the conquest of disease is possible. And it must be brought home to people that the toll taken by disease rises geometrically with the passage of time.

The public have a right to the realistic presentation of goals by the scientific community and to know the prospects for success and the anticipated time to reach different stages of the ultimate goal. Such improved communications soon could be expected to effect congressional and parliamentary attitudes.

So it seems that Canada and the United States face common problems, although Canada has the added burden of loosing highly trained manpower to the United States. Both countries are faced with cutbacks in assistance to biomedical research at a time when it is needed more than ever. Both countries are guilty of not letting the public at large benefit from research findings long since proven. Again, epilepsy is a case in point. Dr. Robb further claimed, "So much can be done for epileptic children if they are treated properly. Yet, a *laissez-faire* attitude prevails. This often means the day-dreaming child is scolded at school and hounded at home." Medical research, operating in a vacuum, has not been integrated and related to the medical education process and with the public's legitimate social goals. In both countries, government and the scientific community have failed to communicate the relevant goals of science and research to an interested public, thereby limiting much needed support. These deficiencies come at a time when new challenges face us in the field of heart disease, cancer, mental illness, slaughter on our highways, arthritis, allergies, the growth of new limbs, to name only a few. More, not fewer, medical scientists must be trained in a host of associated discipline, all of them involved in the business of researching and teaching medicine; biologists, microbiologists, pharmacologists, biomathematicians, biophysicists, biochemists, pathologists. It includes the associated fields of genetics, immunology, anatomy, histology, and clinical medicine.

Could it be that in North America at a time when both Canada and the United States are embarking on massive public schemes of Medicare that many important services won't be there and services that are will slip from excellence to mediocrity. Excellence in research is central to excellence in overall health and medical care services. Yet, right now that lesson is being ignored.

9
The Non-Doctors

Scores of medical people but only a fleeting glimpse of the doctor . . . .

The following account is from the journal entries of a registered nurse. She was working in a British hospital, but her problems are so common to hospitals in North America that they are worthy of inclusion here. The nurse, who had been self-taught in intensive coronary procedures, was in charge of the heart unit in a major city hospital and three other wards. The only help was an "auxiliary," an untrained nursing aide. Beyond the heart unit emergency area, five patients recovering from heart attacks were under observation. Four other patients were suffering from serious conditions. Farther down the passage were two other wards, one containing five seriously ill cancer patients.

> August 17, 1968. 11:45 p.m. – Patient admitted to heart unit with chest pains and an abnormally slow pulse and abnormally high blood pressure. Unable to check and monitor patient. Had to attend a cancer patient who began to hemmorrhage. Auxiliary left to do observation on the heart case.
> Succeeded in stopping the hemmorrhage. Returned to heart unit. Heart case badly deteriorated. Could not observe properly because of other seriously ill patients in wards.
> Three a.m. Cancer patient developed uncontrollable hemmorrhage. Heart patient pulse slowed and blood pressure dropped. Near collapse.

The next day the nurse complained, "Proper coronary observation is impossible under these conditions." The hospital's official reply was, "You are talking a lot of nonsense." and "You are not qualified to comment on hospital procedure."

Night of October 10, 1968 – The general ward situation was the same. Staff now consisted of the nurse with a first-year student nurse. The coronary bay contained two patients in their period of greatest risk on cardiorators (screens which show heartbeats as a moving track of light) and needing, above all, rest, very close observation and freedom from disturbance and excitement.

9:00 p.m. – Advised to expect an attempted suicide by drug overdose. Pointed out that the only beds available were in the coronary bay. Over-ruled. Schizophrenic in a noisy, violent, confused and restless condition admitted to bed next to critically-ill heart patients.

9:30 p.m. – Patient in the coronary bay developed heart stoppage. Called in three night nurses. None knew ward's emergency routine. Coronary patient died.

11:30 p.m. – Semi-collapsed heart case admitted to the last empty bed in the coronary bay. Placed on a cardioratory. Left student nurse to monitor.

Attempted suicide became violent from his overdose. Began jumping in and out of bed, urinating and defecating. Had to try to completely ignore but having very bad effect on heart patients.

Asked the student to do a round of wards. One patient died unnoticed. One of the cancer patients had developed an obstruction and was falling out of bed. Had to leave coronary emergency three times to put patient back in bed. Asked for help. Nurse with no coronary training arrived at 6:30. Dealt with bodies and helped prepare the ward for the day nurse 8:00 a.m.

Not surprisingly, after these and other crisis-filled evenings, the nurse complained again to the management committee. She soon learned that the management officials had little or no knowledge of "technological" nursing and modern medicine.

She said, "There was absolutely no improvement after the meeting. I was given two auxiliaries instead of one; but the first was inefficient even in general nursing procedures and the other was forty years old and six months pregnant."

From the moment someone falls ill or is involved in an accident to the time of recovery, he sees scores of medical people but gets only a fleeting glimpse of the doctor. The rest of the time the patient is in the hands of non-doctors who are loosely referred to as paramedical personnel. The term paramedical applies to those workers in the health field who are endorsed by and work in close association with the medical profession. They comprise all the occupations that have grown up around the healing practitioner.

A limited list of these personnel would read as follows: nurses, laboratory technicians, radiological technicians, medical record librarians, electroencephalography technicians, electrocardiography technicians, physiotherapists, occupational therapists, heart laboratory technicians, assistants in the clinical investigation unit, speech therapists, and rehabilitation nurses.

The term paramedical "departments" as normally used covers three differentiated kinds of activities in the hospital. The largest group are the technicians who staff the laboratories and other diagnostic facilities of the hospital. Next in numerical importance are various kinds of therapists, including the nurse, who provide for patients certain services which lie on the margin of those provided by doctors. The third group provides clerical services handling those hospital records which are distinctly medical in character.

In theory, at least, doctors and paramedical personnel both are parts of a medical team. But, tragically, it rarely works that way.

The first point for specific emphasis is that there is an enormous gap between the two parts of the team. Between doctors and the paramedical occupations there are large differences in income. Doctors start at the top of the income scale in North America. Many of the paramedical personnel are close to the bottom. Both are essential to the practice of medicine, but the rewards and prestige are disproportionately shared. There is no other kind of work in our society where the gap between those who provide a service and those who help is correspondingly wide.

This state of affairs has a direct bearing on recruitment into the paramedical fields. The pool of recruits is meagre. Many of the positions are dominated by unmarried girls with a desire for mobility, and our training facilities for technical people have lagged woefully behind. North American paramedical workers, in general, have no sense of career and they are badly organized.

Training of paramedical people takes little account of the necessity for teamwork, and a large number of today's paramedical personnel are inadequately trained and simply cannot handle modern medical equipment.

It has become imperative that medical personnel be trained in health science centres and that a uniform standard of subsidization for their training be implemented, as well as a proper quality control supervisory system. Obvious as this may be, there is no set of training standards. Some are taught in universities, others in hospitals, yet others by on-the-job training. With small exception, each group trains and eventually operates in a dangerous vacuum.

The health field is shifting away from the pattern of a small, élite medical profession, supplemented by hard-working devoted nurses and other helpers. It is on the way to becoming a mass industry. In order that the industry can be fed by a continuous flow of qualified workers, the same type of career planning and incentives which have been successfully applied in industry must be introduced for paramedical personnel. Above all, it must produce top personnel but without those promotion and financial incentives which are at present ignored, the chances of success are minimal.

There has been token recognition of the desirability of training together the various kinds of health personnel who must later work together, especially in hospital settings. In some instances health science centres are becoming centres of medical regions in a most important way. Medical schools and hospitals with community and regional responsibilities now should have the responsibility of creating a systematic scheme for recruiting, training and deploying the paramedical worker.

Because of her historical and contemporary role on the team, perhaps the best-known member is the nurse. Her importance in the care of the sick is second only, many say equal, to the role of the doctor.

A publication entitled *Nursing Care Plans, a Study Programme in Nursing Management*, and published by the Hospital Continuing Education Project of the Hospital Research and Educational Trust, Chicago, Illinois, lists the expectations of today's trained nurse.

Nursing Objectives on the Surgical Unit

To assist in carrying out the plan for medical care, the nursing staff will:

Maintain close communications with the doctor;
Make certain that the doctor's orders are communicated and carried out promptly;
Assure competent observation, reporting, and recording of physical and vital signs, signs of fluid and electrolyte imbalance, and signs of infection;
Assure correct use, maintenance, and functioning of prescribed equipment;
Assist in plan for rehabilitation.

To facilitate recuperation, thus, the nursing staff will:

Promote maximum independence;
Encourage self-care;
Assist in programme of early ambulation.

To provide bodily care and physical comfort, the nursing staff will:

Assure correct preoperative preparation;
Maintain proper body alignment and positioning of patients in bed;
Assure competent care of surgical dressings, casts, appliances.

To provide emotional support, the nursing staff will:

Help alleviate apprehension about surgery;
Promote positive attitudes toward changes in body function and structure.

To provide a programme of health teaching, the nursing staff will:

Promote good health habits;
Teach self-care;
Reinforce the doctor's instructions.

Obviously a properly trained nurse is a key member of our theoretical team. Through her own initiative she can and does care for the sick and save lives. Yet she is treated as a "poor relation" by the medical profession. Nursing salaries vary widely, but a typical nurse I talked to in Montreal was making $133 per week. The doctors she was working with were making six to ten times that much, a gap both unjustified but typical of the "medical industry."

Let's examine other problems facing the nursing profession. As a by-product of the non-integration of the medical industry, it is obvious there is too much brass at the top. Twenty per cent or 25,000 of Canada's trained registered nurses are doing administrative paperwork amidst a stifling hierarchy which typically runs like this: Superintendent or Director of Nursing; assistant or assistants; Evening Supervisor; Night Supervisor; head nurses; sometimes one or two registered nurses per floor; student nurses and orderlies. Administrative confusion and endless paperwork is a fact of life in nursing today.

Patient-focused nursing care is imperative but can be provided only if nurses are able to turn over non-nursing functions to other departments. The nurse should return to a closer association and contact with the patient. As of now, nurses spend too much time doing unnecessary paperwork, running errands, performing administrative duties, keeping inventory. They can't save lives in an office.

What about communication between the doctor and nurse? Frequently a patient asks the nurse about medication, and about his condition, and blames the nurse for excessive secrecy. The doctor, however, has simply ignored the importance of communication with her. She must navigate in a sea of relative ignorance. The full partnership between physician and nurses too frequently means little more than the handmaiden relationship, which many doctors tend to look upon as an expression of good nursing. In most instances communications between nurses, physicians, medical staff and other departments is deplorable.

The nursing profession is plagued with the same problems that face most other paramedical groups. There is a general failure to establish standards and criteria, including criteria for determining good patient care. Nurses rarely participate in a hospital's budget preparations, there is an unbelievably excessive turnover of personnel, and a dangerously large gap between nursing service and nursing education.

For example, the registered nurse, far too often, cannot handle modern medical equipment. Gloria Gilbert of the Columbia University Department of Nursing says, "Unless medical and nursing schools and in-service education stress the importance of adequate knowledge and understanding of basic electrical principles and safety measures, morbidities and mortalities from electrocution in the hospital will mount."

In Canada, there is no shortage of qualified nurses. There is, however, such a colossal waste of nursing skills from poor utilization of nursing time, turnover of staff, emigration, and non-practicing personnel, that it results in a shortage of available nursing hours.

Unless corrected, the sub-standard levels of salaries and working conditions will, within three or four years, create a crisis in quantity and quality of nurses. Since 1950, in Canada, the percentage of qualified women seeking entry into the profession has declined by 50 per cent. There are, in Canada, approximately 120,000 registered nurses. At first glance we see a healthy ratio of one registered nurse to 164 population, one of the highest in the world. Yet, only half are employed full-time, 19 per cent are employed part-time, 22 per cent are not employed in nursing at all.

Twenty-five to 33 per cent of positions in nursing in Canada require as one qualification a Baccalaureate or higher degree. In actual fact, less than 5 per cent of nurses have these qualifications and the yearly increase of qualified staff is imperceptible. Not surprising, considering the lack of status and financial incentive.

What about turnover? Each year there is a turnover of 61 per cent of the general staff in public general hospitals in Canada. Annually, 40,000 staff nurses change positions. At a cost of $500 per individual change, the total yearly bill is $20,000,000 – the kind of figures that would bankrupt any other major industry, but which is tolerated by those holding the public purse, the medical profession and the public who foot the bill. I asked a number of nurses why they changed jobs and I got some interesting answers. Many were young and single and just wanted to travel, but others said they were frustrated by paperwork and administrative headaches. Others said they wanted to help people, to actually be with patients. Instead, they were counting drugs or running errands for doctors. They were nothing more than water boys on the medical "team."

The nurse is unique. She is the one and only person who can and does attend the patient on a continuous basis. She is a bit of a physician, dietician, physiotherapist and social worker, as well as a primary care giver. In spite of the fact that the nursing profession in North America persists in following traditions, resists innovation, and lacks the personnel to implement change, slowly but surely the changing role of the nurse is evolving. The nurse of tomorrow must take over part of the work-load of the disappearing general practitioner. In a few years she could be responsible for the health care of a group of families in the community and her training must prepare her for that responsibility. The new nurse would move freely from the home to the hospital and back. She would become the family's nurse and her main concern would be health. She will not replace the doctor, but in ten to fifteen years, the practice of nursing must more clearly resemble the practice of the family doctor than that of nursing in the past century. The graduate of the university nursing programme of tomorrow will be a community medical practitioner in the fullest sense of the word. Her responsibility, status and remuneration must be in keeping with that role. Graduates from diploma programmes will largely give care in the hospital and work with the community nurse.

While that should be the direction we are moving in today, all paramedical groups, including nursing, lack trained staff, and the trained staff that we do have is poorly utilized and badly distributed. Moreover, there is little recognition of the urgency of the question on the part of the medical profession and public authorities.

The pattern all over North America is the same. Medicare and Medicaid programmes have been established in many instances and in others they are about to be introduced. Governments and the private sector were forewarned over a decade ago that, unless services were augmented and improved in order to meet the increased demand brought about by voting billions of dollars in the form of income supplementation for health and medical services, the result would be chaos. This chaos would occur not only in the form of skyrocketing costs, but in the form of a near-breakdown in services, by putting a strain on an already outmoded and overburdened non-system. Humane Medicare programmes must ascertain that the services that are meant to be paid for are there in the first place.

The 1967 Report of the Commission of Inquiry on Health and Social Welfare in the Province of Quebec is a progressive and far-reaching document, but its warnings and advice were largely ignored. Nearly four years after the report was published, Quebec introduced Medicare. In the interim, governments both federal and provincial, with the private sector, failed to meet their responsibilities, as outlined in the report, by training more doctors, nurses, and other paramedical workers to meet the challenge of Medicare. The Quebec performance typifies the North American picture and until governments face up to their responsibilities regarding the medical non-system, Medicare will be nothing more than a finance mechanism, a cruel hoax foisted on a confused and disillusioned public and the theoretical "team" will remain theoretical.

10
The Hospital – Part I
Discipline and Control

The question of quality control and discipline involves three basic considerations: standards, surveillance, and enforcement.

The proneness to operate and unnecessarily remove healthy tissue by knife-happy surgeons, as mentioned in Chapter 4, is not offset by proper peer review procedures in most of our hospitals.

In the United States, only 1,350 out of a total of 7,137 hospitals use services for auditing their quality performance provided by the Committee on Professional Hospital Activities. The American Medical Association has consistently opposed any notion of medical auditing and, in particular, they continue to oppose most vehemently the on-site audit aspect of hospital surveillance programmes. In June of 1970, the American Medical Association even rejected proposals by its own special committee to improve health care in the nation and provide consumers with a health "Bill of Rights."

Instead, the Association approved a five-year ten-million-dollar programme on public relations to improve the image of United States' doctors.

In the United States, the accreditation of hospitals was begun in 1918 when the American College of Surgeons compiled a set of minimum standards. Immediately afterwards, it was revealed that more than 85 per cent did not measure up to minimum standards.

In 1969, of the 7,317 voluntary hospitals in the United States, only 4,906 had received "Joint Committee on Accreditation of Hospitals" approval. Yet committee reports are never made public and many internal audit committees never begin to meet committee standards. Moreover, the committee only tests the environment of the hospital and rarely the results of actual treatment.

In the case of private, proprietary hospitals, there is often no method of surveying quality control and staff performance. The rich who go to private, for-profit hospitals, feeling they are exclusive, are frequently subjected to low, uncontrolled standards where the surgery rate is sometimes unnecessarily high.

In North America, far too many accreditation inspection procedures take place only through a voluminous exchange of paperwork between the hospital and the private or public authorities. On-the-site inspection done by qualified personnel is pitifully inadequate. In the United States, accreditation and inspection procedures are next to meaningless and are not uniformly applied across the country. The Joint Commission on Accreditation of Hospitals has the only formal self-regulation programme. Self-regulation means just that. The medical establishment continues to be allowed to regulate itself while remaining aloof from any meaningful public scrutiny. In examining the system of quality control operating within hospitals one finds a general failure by the J.C.A.H. to maintain even their own required standards.

In Canada, the programme of the Canadian Council of Hospital Accreditation attempts to ensure uniform standards of hospital care for all Canadians. Unbelievably, the whole programme is on a voluntary basis. Hospitals which have not requested accreditation often have deplorable standards. Even in so-called accredited hospitals, there is a huge variation in standards. In Canada, the hospital sector has enjoyed amazing immunity from public scrutiny. If, in the future we have the much-needed community and regional clinics to improve the delivery of health and medical services, how can we expect them to be properly controlled and upgraded, when so late in the day, our local hospitals are mostly a law unto themselves? It seems elementary that both in Canada and the United States we need meaningful "national" bodies to operate a mandatory accreditation and inspection programme.

Any examination of North American inspection and accreditation procedures became purely theoretical for the citizens of Montreal in late June, 1970. What the city health department had to say about some of Montreal's most illustrious hospitals, most of which had accreditation, revealed a disgraceful situation.

The Montreal report found standards for the prevention of contagious diseases, air and water pollution and the disposal of waste, including human remains, as falling abysmally short not only of ethical but legal standards. The report criticized careless and undisciplined staff in pathology laboratories and autopsy rooms and made the charge that death certificates were often falsified.

The report also came to the conclusion that the hospitals in question did not meet elementary norms of hygiene in regard to pathology, laboratory and autopsy rooms. Death certificates falsified statistics, particularly by minimizing the number of deaths attributable to contagious disease. The health of the population is threatened, claimed the report, which went on to show how hospital incinerators for waste disposal far from adequately met regulations. The inspectors found it hard to conceal their anger as they outlined conditions in kitchens, wards, rooms, operating rooms, and laundries. Of the rooms and wards of these hospitals, they wrote:

No elementary precautions to follow the simplest rules of hygiene are taken. In those locations where patients have infection or contagious disease, no particular precautions are taken. Waste from treatment, operation, autopsy rooms and labs are frequently wrongly identified. They were often kept in inefficient containers for as long as six weeks, giving off revolting odours. Storage facilities for waste are generally inadequate and insufficient. Incinerators were generally found to be ill-equipped, poorly maintained and inadequately operated, not meeting city by-laws regarding affluents. Handling of hospital waste from all sources was found to be 'unhealthy and dangerous.'

Sometimes the various types of waste were not even kept separate. It speaks of incidents of garbage bags being emptied out on the floor while "their contents are searched for the odd scalpel that may have been lost." The investigating team found conditions particularly bad in pathology labs and autopsy rooms where ventilation was inadequate and "a general state of filthiness resulted from accumulated dust and stained linen, accumulation of unusual objects, dried blood deposits on their floors, floor tiles and walls."

In these rooms the team also noted bad odours, instruments that were "out of date," dirty, covered with blood and rusty, and rooms that have not been cleaned for at least two years. There was also a careless or callous attitude towards human remains which presented a common danger. The investigators recorded:

We deplore the abnormal and dangerous paradox that permits certain members of the medical body to be so negligent with the naked corpses of people who have died of contagious diseases when the same doctors were so meticulous before such a person's death.

75

Although dump inspection was not within investigators' jurisdiction, they went on to report after visiting a city dump:

Sanitary burying is not being done, and no particular precautions are taken with regard to hospital waste.

All kinds of people are permitted to search waste for scavenging. It is obvious that these disposal sites are a source of dissemination of disease and pollution. We were overwhelmed to learn that wastes from many hospitals were disposed of in dumps. We have to conclude, unfortunately, that hospitals generally do not meet elementary hygiene norms.

The authors noted "bad odours, unclean instruments, plumbing submerged under water (danger of polluting water), offensive odours in refrigerated drawers conserving bodies, naked bodies bathed in their blood, and floors that do not have the required shape for directing the liquids to a drain."

On the issue of "erroneous death certificates" the report stated the hospital attitude made it possible to report only 40 per cent of the deaths actually attributable to contagious disease. "It is evident that to falsify statistics contributes to giving the population a false impression of security in regard to these diseases," said the report. The investigators were so stunned and shocked that they considered legal action and criminal charges but they finally concluded:

Infractions are so numerous and so extensive and have so many implications that it was deemed preferable to try to look first for the common solutions before serving legal notice on the institutions concerned. Of course, they added, one would not have to deplore such a situation as exists today had a system of regular inspection been implemented in the past.

The report recommended that pathologists "stop protecting colleagues who sign erroneous death certificates" and that this practice be brought to the attention of the Quebec Health Department.

Moreover, certain government agencies are so deprived of such pertinent information that these agencies cannot envisage a proper programme to control contagious diseases and as a result, the falsification by pathologists risks the life of persons who are called upon to handle corpses.

Communities all over North America have no reason whatsoever to read the Montreal report with any degree of smugness. A survey of most accreditation and inspection procedures has led me to believe Montreal's institutions are the rule and not the exception. At least Montreal health authorities did produce a report. Even then, it was apparently only because of the vigilance and hard work of reporters on the Montreal *Star* that a report was made public. According to later press reports, Victor Goldbloom, a well-known Montreal doctor, and now a Minister in the Quebec government, replied after the report leaked to the public that the way the revelations were made public was regrettable because "they tended to undermine public confidence in the city's hospitals."

Incredible as it may sound, the new Minister said it would have been more beneficial for everyone concerned "if the formulators of the report had sat down with hospital authorities and discussed any deficiencies they may have found before making their findings public."

Goldbloom neglected to specify who "everyone" was and added the even more unfortunate comment, "Public exposure was being done at the expense of public confidence in hospital efficiency."

Doctor Goldbloom can at least be cited for consistency when he terminated with another classic *non sequitur*, "The reputable institutions should have been given an opportunity to make the necessary corrections."

The question of quality control and discipline involves three basic considerations: standards, surveillance, and enforcement.

In the area of hospitals, both in Canada and the United States, public national authorities must be made responsible for the adequate staffing and financing of accreditation programmes. Hospitals failing to obtain accreditation would be meticulously examined by state or provincial authorities who would be ultimately responsible for following up each individual case and for determining whether or not the hospital in question should be allowed to continue in operation.

Regarding the disciplining of the profession itself, the province of Quebec has surely taken the lead in this regard. The Castonguay report recommends that all professions, including medicine, law, architecture, and engineering would be submitted to the same general rules, making professional associations into public bodies supervised jointly by the government and universities. Regulations adopted by various professional associations would have to be debated in public before being given approval by the government.

In developing standards of optimal care, university medical centre clinics and hospitals should often be considered as centres where excellence is encouraged.

If "peer review" and medical auditing is to be made meaningful, medical record procedures must be updated with the help of computer technology.

Above all, we must ask what is the answer to the following questions? Can the maintenance of quality standards and the disciplining of physicians be left with the medical profession? Can the North American public feel sure that their doctors are reasonably up to date on diagnostic and treatment techniques? Does the physician and hospital keep such records so that at a later date work can be evaluated and will the doctor's work, no matter where performed, be monitored, objectively, with reasonable frequency?

11
The Hospital – Part II
A Place To Die

... the impersonality of a place where people are dying among strangers. —GEORGE ORWELL

In Canada and the United States, as recently as the last century, hospitals were supported by charity and were often referred to as "pesthouses," places for the penniless sick. Because of the great danger of infection in the pesthouses, the rich were cared for in their homes. As the years passed, modern hospitals have supposedly been transformed into citadels of science where diagnosis, treatment, and preventative medicine constitute the basis of their activities.

Of the approximately 8,000 hospitals of various types we have in North America the voluntary community hospitals are, in many ways, the most important. Certainly they are the most important in relation to advanced medical technology and skills. Today, four out of ten hospital beds in North America are in tax-free, voluntary institutions, receiving both paying and non-paying cases. Unfortunately, at the voluntary community hospital level, the many advances in the art of medicine have not been matched by similar advances in hospital organization, efficiency, economics, administration, and management techniques. At best, their economics are makeshift while waste, duplication, administrative laxity, and inefficiencies piled on inefficiencies plague what has been accurately described as our hospital non-system.

A great number of people have come to look upon the modern hospital as the central institution in the delivery of medical and health services. If this is so, it is here that we find the administrative chaos and managerial breakdown that plague the non-system in the delivery of North American medical and health care. In many hospitals I investigated, more drugs were thrown out than used because of a lack of inventory or stock control. Certain drugs lose their effectiveness after a definite period and have a specific "life expectancy or shelf time." No attempts were made to come to terms with these facts. The costly waste was incredible and often could not be measured.

Voluntary hospitals today are being directed, not managed, much

79

as they were at the turn of the century. When it comes to running them, we are truly using horse-and-buggy methods in the computer age.

The medical professionals have been inordinately slow to make use of modern techniques. Doctors have clearly misunderstood the benefits which could be introduced by modern computer technology, feeling it would lessen their personal influence and, at times, dehumanize medical practice. In all fairness, they are not alone in that. Let us look at one example. Patient care is entirely dependent upon the accumulation and analysis of information. Physician decisions are normally contingent upon the results of such tests as laboratory, X-Ray, electrocardiogram, and isotope. Usually, twenty-four hours exist between the moment the physician decides to order a series of diagnostic procedures and the time he receives the results. Definite treatment waits upon these results. The time involved in the most lengthy diagnostic processes seldom exceeds one hour, and more often the procedures involve only a matter of minutes. What about the balance of the twenty-four to forty-eight-hour waiting period? Often it is plagued with paperwork and the circulation of information long since made obsolete by the computer. First of all the doctor writes the order. The order is then transcribed on to the patient's chart, then on to a lab request. The request is then transferred to the lab by messenger or tube. The lab technician is then dispatched to obtain a specimen, and returns to the lab, where the test is processed and the results recorded. The results are then filed in the patient's chart. The physician completing his office hours reaches the hospital and studies the information. Basic computer technology and hospital scheduling programmes could have rectified this time-consuming procedure years ago. Yet, with a few exceptions, there is no general evidence that those who could bring about the changes, doctors, are beginning to even think about it. The results of not utilizing modern computer technology and managerial techniques were predictable. The trend toward shorter hospital stays brought about by advanced medical knowledge has been reversed and the average stay in North American community hospitals is 8.4 days, one day longer than six years ago.

Accounting methods are another factor to consider. They are often antiquated at best, and in the vast majority of North American community hospitals the most elementary accounting methods were only introduced with the advent of Medicare and Medicaid programmes. Many voluntary hospitals kept and still keep their books secret, entrusting hit-or-miss bookkeeping procedures to overworked nurses.

Today, every fourth North American family is affected, annually, by a hospital admission, and hospital doors are open to everyone even if, at times, this theory is not borne out in practice. The increased demand for hospital services, stimulated by insurance coverage, and superimposed on a relatively static supply of hospital facilities, has seriously hampered the quality of our hospital care. Add to this the outmoded managerial techniques now largely employed to run our hospitals and the predictable result is chaos.

No subject, within the hospital sector, gets more play than the topic of regional hospital planning. In effect, the question has assumed such importance and meaning that Canada's Minister of National Health and Welfare, John Monroe, threatened to impose regional hospital and health planning by government control and compulsion unless such an end could be attained by voluntary means. The Minister declared,

> Let me state plainly that it is my feeling that if the hospitals and other health facilities in this country will not get together to coordinate their services and divide their specialized functions, then my provincial colleagues and I will have to give serious thought to the selective use of government funds to foster this goal ourselves.

What is regional hospital planning?

It involves the notion that hospitals are (at least) partially responsible for the health and medical needs of the particular community in which they find themselves. To meet community needs for high-quality care, and to meet them in a humane and economic way, there must be planning. And the planning must be aimed at meeting these needs and not at simply fostering the growth of the hospital as is often the case. People must come first.

The majority of hospital boards and administrators all over North America go through the motions of acknowledging the principle of regional planning. They employ consultants who make population forecasts, conduct patient-origin studies, analyze utilization experience, and so on. What invariably happens is that the programme of expansion usually passed by the board for state or provincial approval reflects merely the needs of the community, as subjectively determined by the department heads of the hospital. The surgeon, the paediatrician, the radiologist, the internist, and others submit their "wants." The total want list then forms the basis for the hospital's expansion programme. Only by the rarest set of circumstances are real community needs ever reflected. Almost always, institutional growth is considered in the rarified atmosphere of "what is most convenient and best for the medical profession." Departmental empire-building hardly ever reflects the legitimate demands of community need.

Individual hospitals, emphasizing institutional prestige and empire-building, have no idea of community or regional needs in relation to services and the number of beds required in the areas of intensive care, intermediate care, self-care, long-term care, and organized home care. Also distorting the picture is the lack of properly staffed regional and community clinics. Many of our community hospitals have their origins in specific religious organizations. As praiseworthy as many of their activities were and are, a major preoccupation has not been with the overall needs of the community at large.

Most North American hospitals are orientated toward curative treatment of established disease at an advanced or critical stage. In many hospitals, over half their admissions take place through the emergency units, clearly demonstrating the low priority given to preventive treatment in our communities. Also, because of the largely impersonal care given in some of our vast hospital complexes, there is little or no patient followup once he is discharged. As Michael Crichton recently wrote, "The hospital can no longer act as a stronghold of technological, scientific excellence for a few patients when the disparity between patient marvels and community horrors is ever increasing." His thinking is seconded by Dr. John Knowles of the Massachusetts General Hospital who claims that hospitals must give up "the present defensive isolation . . . in a bastion of acute, curative, specialized and technical medicine."

In both Canada and the United States, adequate public and private expenditures could do much to reduce hospital admissions. If proper priority were given to expenditures for preventive medicine, health care centres, general ambulatory care centres, home care programmes, regional and community clinics, nursing and convalescent homes, and other facilities that could treat and care for patients who now find themselves admitted to general community hospitals, much could be done to bring order into the near breakdown of hospital services which is now taking place. Knowles feels far too much emphasis is put on the hospital's record and performance after the patient has gone through its doors. He states that admissions from the impoverished areas of inner cities would decline by 80 per cent if more effort were spent in preventing diseases and sickness in the first place. Hospitals of the future, amongst other things, must be the base for comprehensive community services extending their expertise and resources into the community. Such is not the case today.

It is true that regional and community planning of hospital facilities requires a high degree of organized local self-initiative. On the other hand, communities cannot do this by themselves unless there is some order at the top. Mr. Monroe's threat from Ottawa was fine, but both Ottawa and Washington would do well to put their own houses in order before lecturing to state, provincial and local governments. Common to both federal establishments in the early 1970's is an unbelievable state of absolute chaos in relation to welfare programmes. Health and medical services must surely lead the parade of confusion, lack of controls, duplication and waste. It is very odd to hear federal officials lecturing on these issues at the community level, while Ottawa and Washington consistently refuse to clarify and define health and medical care goals, and to give integration and direction to their programmes. Their fragmentary approach merely encourages disorder at the local level. Much of the confusion results from both federal governments bowing far too frequently to the prestigious medical lobbies which have kept overly-sensitive politicians on tenterhooks far too often. In both countries, official advisory boards and agencies have continually warned those empowered to act on the true nature of community needs. But little has happened.

During the Depression years, and for the duration of the Second World War, few hospitals were constructed and for this reason many hospitals in the United States and Canada became obsolete and there were extreme shortages in the number of hospital beds and related hospital facilities. Consequently, on August 13, 1946, Congress enacted into law the Hill-Burton programme with the passage of the *Hospital Survey and Construction Act*. The purpose of the Act was to survey needs and to assist the local sponsors in the several states in the construction of public and other non-profit hospitals. The Hill-Burton programme dominated hospital construction in the past, even though its grants bore only about 15 per cent of construction costs.

When we look at Washington's example, we should not be too optimistic about the central government taking any dynamic lead in the area of community or regional planning. While the Hill-Burton programme is the main federal initiative in hospital construction, seven uncoordinated federal programmes for hospital construction are invariably responsible for waste and duplication at the local level. The Office of Economic Opportunity, Commerce's Economic Development Administration, The Small Business Administration, amongst other agencies, often intervene at the local level without any idea of what other agencies of the state or federal governments are doing.

Take, for example, the situation in one Florida city. The city of Belle Glade, Florida is a small rural community in the state's southern interior. In February, 1963, the Hill-Burton programme approved a grant of $635,000 in federal funds toward the construction of a new $1.6 million, 75-bed hospital. This hospital was completed in 1965 and now has an occupancy rate of between 50 and 55 per cent. On average, little more than half of the beds in the hospital are used. In August, 1965, the month before the Glade's Memorial Hospital opened, the Small Business Administration approved a $60,000 loan to the Carver Memorial Hospital Holding Corporation to build a 13-bed hospital in Belle Glade. Two years later, the same corporation received approval for an additional $10,000 from the s.b.a. Carver Memorial Hospital was not necessary, and administrators of the Small Business Administration were advised of this by State of Florida health officials.

Even when expenditures are confined to one federal department we have no guarantee for common sense. An example is to be found in the San Francisco Bay area. The Army and Navy refused to consolidate into one joint facility the separate hospitals each were planning to build. The General Accounting Office of the federal government and private hospital planners in the area recommended a joint facility be built and shared by each service. The services refused. They said there was a strong preference on the part of military personnel to be treated in a hospital of their own service. Planning authorities pointed out that medical training and treatment would have been upgraded in a larger facility, but this did not deter the military, and the taxpayers are paying dearly. The General Accounting Office estimated that before the hospitals were built ten million dollars would be wasted with the construction of two separate facilities. Furthermore, the G.A.O. said an additional $8.2 million would be wasted each year from the maintenance and operation of two separate hospitals.

Construction of hospitals has been disorganized and haphazard.

84

Archaic and bad architectural design in many hospitals has led to inefficiencies and waste that industry would not have tolerated in the nineteenth century. Some experts go so far as to state that from the point of view of design and planning, modern hospitals invariably make psychological demands that may retard recovery, casting the patient into a strange, impersonal and alien atmosphere more suited to doctors' demands than to patients' needs.

When discussing hospital construction, we are faced with a real paradox. On the one hand, in the United States and Canada, we must spend eight billion dollars to modernize the existing plant and some three and a half billion dollars for some hundred thousand additional beds in poorly serviced communities. Because of poor regional planning, there is a critical shortage of hospital beds in some areas, but generally speaking our hospitals are under-utilized. Inventories of regional needs are rarely taken, while organized admission and discharge procedures are mostly non-existent. This means that of the approximately 900,000 beds in North American general hospitals, 20 per cent are always empty.

In many ways, the rapidly rising costs and increasing inefficiencies for health care in hospitals is due to the undercapitalization of service plant. Funds for modernization, renovation, and replacement are woefully insufficient. In Canada and the United States, Medicare programmes were meant to mean more social justice, but rarely, if ever, were they implemented before consultation with hospital authorities. Ottawa and Washington were preoccupied with voting money for free services, but paid next to no attention to ascertain whether or not the services were available to buy. The programmes were voted long before initial plans were made to ready proper hospital facilities and things are getting worse. In the latest United States federal budget, 12.3 billion dollars were allotted to income supplementation for medical care, while only three hundred and sixty-one million dollars have been provided for the construction and modernization of hospitals.

Ottawa's slashing of the Health Resources Fund has also had an alarming effect. Once more, the province of Quebec and the Castonguay Commission Report typify only too well the North American scene. Over four years ago, this report concluded that regional planning was a number one priority in any progressive public Medicare plan. At the centre of each region, concluded the report, should be found a large health-training centre, with university affiliation, together with a large teaching hospital which should include all highly specialized services. Decentralized from this large unit, often to be found in smaller towns, cities, and suburbs, the Castonguay committee recommended the establishment of general hospitals of over 200 beds where general surgery and some specialized functions could be performed. Further decentralization, under Castonguay's plan, should see the establishment of hospitals for the care of chronic diseases, old people's and nursing homes, ambulatory care centres, convalescent homes, health care clinics and so on. In effect, Ottawa obliged the provinces to participate in a universal Medicare plan, but voted meaningless sums to help them make ready the plant, facilities and personnel needed under the new programmes. Quebec is no exception. Regions all over North America have embarked on Medicare programmes before services were prepared. The disgraceful results are yet to be seen.

Hospitals cannot raise the money required either from government grants or private subscription to meet the demands of modernization for their facilities. Their inefficiencies are compounded as they hobble along on antiquated equipment. The Royal Edward Chest Hospital in Montreal, for example, is badly in need of funds for new equipment in order to enable certain departments to operate much more efficiently and economically.

Waste and duplication is easily detected in relation to some highly complicated hospital operations. In 1967, 776 u.s. hospitals maintained facilities for open heart surgery. Thirty-one per cent of them did not use their capacity for over a year. In New York City, twenty hospitals were equipped to perform open heart surgery, but only five did two-thirds of all the operations. This does not only involve considerations of waste, but means operating personnel get dangerously rusty for complicated surgery in under-utilized open heart surgery units.

While hospitals are not businesses in the usually accepted sense of the word, it is easy to see that the refusal of most North American hospital authorities to incorporate sound business and management principles into their direction could soon spell the complete end of their usefulness in our health and medical care delivery system. Consider the suburban hospital which absolutely had to have a two-million-volt X-Ray machine, costing $200,000 to buy and install for treating cancer patients and then used it only fifty times a year. Consider the billing clerks who never know when a billing slip gets "lost," since they rely on the nurses to prepare and the messengers to deliver them.

Consider the small hospital which purchased a third-generation computer it couldn't afford, couldn't staff properly, and couldn't get to do half the things the salesman said it could do. The majority of hospitals in a region would do well to share one well-staffed computer. Instead, most hospitals in a specific region have no computer, and those that do more often than not buy a machine before they have begun to train staff to use it. Community hospitals in a region, instead of sharing high-cost facilities, individually purchase expensive equipment which remains woefully under-utilized.

Both in Canada and the United States, insurance plans of all kinds, including Medicare and Medicaid, have truly damaged hospital care and service. Far too often they only include in-patient hospital services, neglecting coverage for out-patient charges. Most plans encourage doctors to hospitalize patients who should not be and many studies have already shown doctors to be notoriously hospital-prone. Private doctors practicing on a fee for service basis in Sault Ste. Marie, Ontario, put their patients into hospital 25 per cent more often than salaried doctors in the same city, according to a study by the United Steelworkers of America. The study involved 23,000 patients in two groups. The private fee for service doctors were responsible for double the rate of hospital admissions, for respiratory diseases, 36 per cent more hospital surgery, and three times the number of tonsil and adenoid removals.

Outdated hospital management techniques perhaps have their most serious implications in relation to personnel. Generally, it can be concluded that hospital management has been left behind by modern techniques which means nurses and other paramedical staff are suffering from a generation gap. The gap has come about because management are generally members of a generation who were trained and spent their formative years in paramedical work before the advent of modern medical machinery. They don't try to understand heart machines and often detest the "dehumanizing" metal boxes with their knobs and dials. This has resulted in millions and millions of dollars of valuable medical equipment lying unused around North American hospitals because of untrained staff. Many new hospitals are relatively useless because new equipment can't be handled by personnel. Unkind as it may sound, we cannot wait five or ten years for the passage of time to replace those who cannot cope with change. If we do, things will quickly get worse. Hospital service will collapse, surrounded by the debris of an era it does not understand. These conditions mean lives are lost that could be saved, and that the unskilled handling of routine equipment often snuffs out the lives of those who are admitted to hospital in a relatively healthy condition.

For years, hospitals depended on and exploited low-cost labour. Today, all over North America, strikes are common everyday features of the hospital scene. The wage demands of North America's two million six hundred thousand hospital employees should be no cause for surprise. Hospital employees, in general, used to rank among the most underpaid workers in the continent. In parts of the southern United States, they earned as little as thirty-five cents per hour. Unions began entering the field in the United States and Canada in the late fifties. Then came a series of bitter strikes. No longer could hospital authorities play on the sympathies of workers because health care was involved. Altruism was one thing. Eating three square meals a day was another. In the United States, federal minimum wage laws were belatedly introduced into the hospital field in 1967. Billions of new federal funds from Ottawa and Washington have flowed into the hospital sector, while resistance to the unions has collapsed. In the years 1966 to 1969, the minimum wage in New York City went from $69.00 a week to $100.00. Non-union hospitals have been obliged to follow suit because of the increasing shortages of trained people, including paramedical aides of all types. Labour leader Jean J. Davis, led a hard-hitting battle for better hospital wages and working conditions. A Russian-born pharmacist, he went to jail for a month in 1962 for refusing to call off a strike. His union now has 42,500 members in 150 hospitals in the New York area alone.

Labour and personnel relations in hospitals are at least thirty years behind most of the other parts of our labour economy, and because of the unbusinesslike methods of hospital management, no group suffers as much as "personnel." As a result, there has been no increase, and very probably a decrease, in hospital "productivity" over the past few years.

What about overall productivity? Productivity in a hospital does not merely mean more efficiency in costs, it also means a steady improvement in standards of health and medical care. Over the past twenty years there is absolutely no evidence that labour productivity has made any advance in North American hospitals, although during the same period in the United States, output per unit of labour in the economy as a whole has advanced at 3.3 per cent a year.

The average size of our community hospitals is another fact which pin-points our non-planning approach to the hospital sector, and accounts in part for its dismal productivity record. Of course, in sparsely settled rural areas there is often little or no choice in determining the size of a community hospital. Yet even in these cases, one well placed central hospital could and should replace two or three tiny, inefficiently run units. One central 200-bed hospital, the hub of regional, medical and health care needs, which would mean properly staffed clinics in the outlying rural areas, is often preferable to five scattered 50-bed hospitals. The average size of all hospitals in the United States is 233 beds. This includes psychiatric hospitals, which average 1,300 beds. The average size of United States' community hospitals is 135 beds. In the critical community hospital industry, the basic unit of product is quite small. For the community hospital industry as a whole, 58.8 per cent of the hospitals have less than 100 beds, 78.8 per cent have less than 200 beds. Only 3.2 per cent are considered to be large hospitals – having over 500 beds. Investigations have shown that the smaller the hospital, the lower the occupancy rate. These hospitals are committed to operate at low and inefficient levels. What about standards? The smaller the hospital, the fewer the facilities and services. Only 12 per cent of United States hospitals with less than twenty-five beds provide a pathology laboratory, whereas, 100 per cent of hospitals with over 500 beds have this facility. The same is true for accreditation, for whatever it may be worth. Less than one per cent of hospitals with fewer than 25 beds are accredited by the American Hospital Association, while 37 per cent of those with 25 to 49 beds, and 75 per cent of those with 50 to 99 beds are accredited. It must be added, though, that accreditation by the American Hospital Association is no guarantee of good quality treatment and care in large hospitals.

It must be repeated, ability to organize has been a major factor in the advance of North American industry. Planning, which can be considered as an integral part of organization, is rapidly becoming perhaps the most important element in the industrial system. Lack of planning in our hospital sector has meant a badly motivated labour force due to poor working conditions, low wages, obsolete and sometimes non-existent channels of promotion. The result has been a decline in productivity and a shameful lowering of health and medical care standards at a time when medical scientists have made breakthroughs in knowledge for the supposed benefit of all North Americans.

Hospitals have the primary responsibility of providing quality health care which, in the past, has too often precluded effective business management. The recent explosion in medical technology and the escalating cost of hospital labour have brought dramatic increases in operating expenses, which make the application of modern business techniques even more essential.

Unfortunately, hospitals have always suffered from a dichotomy of operating philosophies – the lives/dollars problem – which has created a communications gap between the business and professional sides of hospital activity. This gap must be bridged if the dramatic hospital cost spiral is to be controlled. The keys to bridging the gap, from the financial manager's point of view, are understanding, imagination, and the effective use of business techniques. Some of the broad categories of business management which must be applied to hospitals are staff organization and effective communication, meaningful financial reporting, regional planning and sharing of high-cost facilities, effective utilization of manpower, increased utilization of available capacity, and computer technology.

Hospital authorities must start asking basic questions such as:

Can patients who require relatively little care be segregated in lightly staffed, low-cost nursing stations? Is radioisotope and cobalt therapy equipment used in "commercial" quantities? Can sharing agreements be effected with neighbouring hospitals? Is surgery scheduled during morning hours only?

We cannot expect the rate of change in the art and technology of medical practice to decrease. Indeed we can be certain that it will increase at a faster and faster rate. If hospital management techniques do not meet the challenge of change, the North American public will be cruelly and unnecessarily deprived of the benefits of recent advances.

Although it comes from an ancient tradition, the modern North American hospital as we know it today is not much more than forty years old. In another eight years or so we shall hardly be able to recognize today's hospital. Its services will be confined to those cases which truly require hospitalization, and it will cease to be a convalescent facility. With more emphasis placed on the hospital's community role, the hospital of tomorrow will play a larger part in the area of preventative medicine. It will seek out people who need hospitalizaion but are not receiving it, and will treat others so that their future hospitalization will be prevented. Tomorrow's teaching hospitals will use television and computers to spread new research information far beyond their doors, as medical education reaches outside their walls.

Many of the particular problems facing our hospitals are common to any general discussion of the whole field of North American health and medical services. Our highly fragmented approach to the delivery of these services is doubly true when we talk about hospitals. There is no integrated approach, definition of goals, or co-operation between levels of government; between the public or private sectors or, in either country, between separate departments or agencies within the federal establishment. It is this set of circumstances that so often makes the necessary regional or community planning of hospital resources next to impossible.

It was George Orwell who said, "In every hospital death, there will be some cruel, squalid detail, perhaps too small to be told but leaving painful memories behind, arising out of the haste, the crowding, the impersonality of a place where every day people are dying among strangers."

Surely this can be changed.

12
The Hospital – Part III
The Non-System!

Arguing against the medical staff when they want some-thing in this hospital is like arguing against motherhood.
HOSPITAL ADMINISTRATOR

At present the hospital industry is the third or fourth largest in North America and by 1975 the health services industry will be the number one employer in both Canada and the U.S. When we consider such massive spending, combined with something as important as the health and well-being of our people, it would be easy to assume that in the hospital sector we could find a high level of central authority, which possessed real direction and purpose. Yet hospitals continue to remain a law unto themselves, and the opposite is more often the case. Most hospitals are normally *mis*directed by a loose triumvirate, the board of governors, the administrator, and the medical staff, usually working at odds in separate vacuums, and spurred on to conflicting goals by overlapping and blurred lines of authority and jurisdiction.

One typical case involving a large Montreal hospital immediately comes to mind. In this instance, the board of governors resembled community hospital boards all over the continent, its members being mostly heads of large business or financial concerns or community leaders in other fields. The hospital was engaged in a large expansion programme and the board was trying to decide how many elevators would be needed in the multi-storied building. Architects and planners strongly recommended a certain number, having made projections based on thorough investigations. Then they put their case to the board which was faced with realistic budget limitations. At this point, the doctor representing the medical staff strongly vetoed any idea that so many elevators were needed. He argued, quite correctly from his point of view, that the money would be better spent on much needed modern lab equipment.

The outcome was that the architects and planners were overruled. A year after the expansion was completed, waits for elevators were so long that hospital efficiency was seriously impaired as exasperated crowds of staff, visitors, and even patients backed up down the halls. Soon the order went out for more elevators. The spectacle of demolition workers tearing down the centre of a modern hospital with all its high cost in-put was enough to give any cost engineer a lifetime of sleepless nights. This particular fiasco wasted over two million dollars, and typifies the kind of authority medical staff have over the running of our hospitals. More often than not, their authority dominates the administrator whose powers are so limited that he administers in theory alone, and it dominates the well-meaning and public spirited "volunteer" board, whose individual members would never, in most instances, contemplate implementing such decisions in the businesses or other institutions they run in the community. Members of the board of governors as well as administrators themselves rarely feel qualified to question the specialized needs and demands of doctors and so the medical staff have an undue influence over our hospital industry. Moreover, many administrators are themselves doctors, with little or no managerial know-how. One administrator told me: "Arguing against medical staff when they want something is like arguing against motherhood."

Most business directors demand clear explanations from management before business decisions are arrived at, especially in areas of high expertise which are often surrounded with the verbiage of the "specialist." Doctors rarely have to account to anybody except other doctors. Boards of governors take them at their word and, together with the administrator, rubber-stamp decisions they would never even entertain in their own world of business. Administrators, trustees and governors must often feel as I did during my first year as a member of parliament sitting on the Estimates Committee of The House of Commons. This committee is responsible for examining the estimated expenditures of government, department by department. On one particular day, a naval Rear-Admiral was testifying before the committee on the cost of a submarine chaser-type destroyer. The estimated cost of the ship was in the neighbourhood of four million dollars. By the time it was completed, the Canadian taxpayer had a bill of around eighteen million dollars. The admiral dutifully explained to us that technological advances during construction necessitated many design changes and thus the necessity for soaring costs. Under questioning by the committee, the admiral, rather than resorting to clear language and clear answers, somehow or other conveyed the impression he wasn't very impressed with the patriotism of members of parliament who seemed overly concerned with dollars and cents when the defence of freedom was involved. Hospital administrators, trustees, and governors are, likewise, made to feel at a disadvantage with medical staff when matters of life and death are being discussed. There seems to be an impression in the medical establishment that any great emphasis on organization, control, efficiency and costs, infringes on the quality of health and medical care, that somehow or other efficiency and high standards of care are incompatible.

The Canadian and American Medical Associations are correct in their emphasis on high standards and a high quality of health and medical services, but until they become much more involved in the efficiency, organization and cost of services, we shall continue to be faced with the fact that doctors, individually and collectively, have for too long ignored their responsibilities in the area of organization. Their "Pavlovian dog" reaction to considerations of efficiency has seriously imperilled their effectiveness. Doctors will always be central figures in any modern team involved in delivering services. Without their co-operation and enthusiastic support, nothing much can be done. Yet, too often, taken as a group they perform as individual entrepreneurs working in a vacuum in our hospitals, demanding instant respect. Society can no longer tolerate such an attitude.

Fortunately times are changing. No longer are doctors held in instant awe by an army of underpaid lackeys ready to jump at their every command. Every other modern professional has long since learned this lesson. Certainly modern business managers and executives have. The era of the "I'm always right" president who instilled the fear of God into the employees went out of the window with silent movies. This doesn't always mean "decision by committee" but it often means decisions by one man who has learned to work and co-operate with others on a team. When doctors try to run hospitals they are not practicing medicine, and this is happening too often today.

Analogies are always dangerous to make. Yet, we must know that a perennial 300-hitter in baseball helps to fill his club's stadium and make a profit for management as well as helping his team win games. He's a central figure in the success story. Let the same player take over the front executive office and try running the entire team-stadium effort, and his batting average and club profits would soon plummet, to say nothing about the loss of games. By insisting on dominating hospitals' front offices, too many doctors are forgetting how to practice medicine. Their administrative bumbling has resulted in such inefficiencies and chaotic control at the hospital level that if continued they will sadly and cruelly nullify many of the benefits modern medical advances and discoveries should have long since been conferred on all the peoples of North America.

In the business and industrial community, we have fortunately passed the period when primary stress was on profit. Not only does the approach mean dehumanization, but it also means ultimate failure. Executives who haven't learned this by now are liable to lose their jobs. Modern, progressive business leaders have long since become aware of the creative advantages in the team approach, the inter-relationship of efficiency and humanism, of profits and real progress. Hospitals are not, of course, industrial concerns in the accepted sense of the word. On the other hand, the outright hostility of the medical establishment to everything sound business practice means and has learned over the years, together with short-sighted and stupid government policies, is largely responsible for the present hospital shambles.

Hospital administrators must administer, governors must govern, doctors must practice. It is a sad commentary on the vast majority of our North American community hospitals that the medical staff invariably feel that the myth must be perpetuated; and any meaningful powers for the administrator and any significant decisions taken by the board would mean their time-honoured empire would come crumbling down. Instead of administrators, we have harassed referees. Instead of responsible board meetings, we have indifferent *pro forma* rubber-stamping. Instead of doctors practicing with the co-operation of and co-operating with good managerial and policy know-how offered by men and women equally dedicated as they, we have doctors part-time doctoring and part-time administering and doing neither particularly well.

An examination of the board, the administration and the medical staff gives discouraging insight. Theoretically speaking, at the policy-making level we find the board of trustees. In the past, when many of our community hospitals depended on local fund raising drives and local donations for financing, individual trustees were largely recruited on the basis of their ability to raise funds. It was also relatively clear what policy-making authority they had. Relatively clear, that is, in relation to the present state of affairs. Today, community hospitals receive almost all their funds from government, diminishing the importance of local bequests and fund-raising. Governments, when allocating funds, often dictate both directly and indirectly broad policy questions for the hospitals concerned. These two facts greatly alter the role of the board of trustees, but, unfortunately, this is rarely recognized. Not sure what they are meant to be doing, trustees collectively and individually interfere in complex administrative matters. This means policy decisions are delayed or not made and results in operational nightmares. Realistically, the board can only concern itself with a few responsibilities: to see that competent people are appointed to key positions, to see that they are fired if they prove incompetent, to insist on controls that measure progress or lack of it, and to see that the hospital meets the needs of the community. All over North America, community hospital trustees with exceptional individual talent are rarely assigned jurisdiction over policy areas which correspond to their particular expertise.

What about the administrator? Ideally speaking, the hospital administrator should do just that – run the hospital. It rarely happens that way. Too often the medical staff have the ear of the trustees to the disadvantage of the administrator's proper function. Crowded by medical staff on the one hand and interfered with by trustees on the other, administrators are given responsibilities without the power to carry them out.

In the past, administrators were often physicians who wanted to slow down but more often now, hospital administration is becoming a field for bright young men. Several universities conduct graduate and post-graduate programmes in the field, but professional hospital administrators are still relatively scarce. Hospitals need more of these men, men who are learned in their organization's product without having or needing M.D. diplomas on the wall; men who talk the hospital language to the physician without condescension on either side; men who can apply business methods to medical matters with full consideration of the medical responsibility and without sounding like automatons. One area in which North America has been consistently the most competent is in the field of industrial management. It is about time we started to manage our hospital industry.

Finally, we have doctors and medical staff. Not always but almost always they dominate the management and policy directives of our hospitals. They are not qualified to handle the job. They largely control internal procedures, admissions and discharges, length of stay, the ordering of tests and drugs, and by their continued opposition to modern paramedical training, they carry the major responsibility for the archaic and outmoded personnel setups that plague North American hospital efficiency. Consider the chief of medical services who refuses to have an extended conversation with any of the administrative people in his hospital, except with the lay administrator in board meetings, to whom he then says, "You don't understand anything about health care! How can you bother me about costs when I deal in lives?" Often the administrator must insist that members of the medical staff who are trustees complete their medical records, or he may have to insist that they report unexpected deaths to the coroner. When, as is sometimes the case, the medical staff in question are members of the governing board and the administrator is not, things can become more than a little delicate. It seems that, through some colossal blunder, we have allowed doctors as private entrepreneurs to have great influence and authority in the affairs of "the corporation." It is the direct cause of many of our administrative problems. Control in many areas is duplicated by the administrator and the physician. This means that hospital workers take orders which are frequently in conflict. The lines of communications and organizational control are unclear and ambiguous. The result is confusion on the part of the hospital worker, and conflict and inefficiency in the hospital environment.

The control and rule of the doctors has become almost impossible in some isolated areas. Doctors are hard to recruit in such communities, and they get their way by threatening to quit.

The common myth about the organizational structure of the community hospital goes something like this. Medical activities are directed by a medical director, and administrative activities by the administrator. These two men are on the same level and are indirectly responsible to one another. They both report to a governing body of responsible citizenry which makes all policy decisions. Under the medical director are the chief of medical staff, the chief of surgical staff, the chief residents, active staff, courtesy staff, residents and interns. Responsible to the administrator are the director of nursing, chief dietitian, and assistant administrators for services and management.

There are hospitals in which this form of organization probably does apply, but only in a very small percentage. The structure is really only applicable to large teaching hospitals, less than 3 per cent of the total number of community hospitals. Even in this small group there are several important discrepancies. The first of these is that the administrator is seldom on a level equivalent to the medical director. Invariably the governing body will back the medical director in disputes. Dr. Sidney Lee described the situation well by saying that the doctors play golf with the board of trustees, but the administrator does not. The social gulf between doctors and "others" pervades the hospital non-system.

In many ways, this is the typical community hospital. There is no medical director and medical staff. The physicians associated with the hospital are all from the group innocuously referred to in the organization chart as "courtesy staff." These are private physicians who have staff privileges at a particular hospital. The physician dominates the hospital environment. He has the authority and the power and an easy access to the board of trustees. Although not part of the organization, and not responsible to it, he makes virtually all decisions involving the expenditures of money, and justifies his authority on the basis of maintaining quality of care. This is, of course, a valid argument but its impact must be weighed against other considerations.

Take the case of the lady in a community hospital for observation. After admission, five or six tests were completed over a forty-eight-hour period, after which she sensed there were no more to come. Two days went by and nobody came near her room except the lady who carried in her meals and a floor nurse who appeared to take her temperature at regular intervals. The lady felt something had gone wrong and went to the head floor nurse to inquire about being discharged. "Who's your doctor?" inquired the nurse. The patient told her. The nurse made some inquiries and found the doctor in question had gone to a convention in Chicago. "You'll have to wait till he returns at the end of the week," said the nurse. The patient continued to plead, and eventually the nurse phoned the doctor's associate in a downtown office who, in turn, contacted Chicago. One hour later the lady was discharged.

Doctors commit large sums of money whenever they treat a patient in a hospital. Too frequently, they fail to recognize and accept responsibilities for the financial implications of their activities. An admission to hospital should only be requested in the context of a clearly-defined purpose and previously thought out plan. Our community hospitals rarely have an organized approach to pre-admission, active treatment and investigation or discharge planning. Prior to the admission of an elective patient, unless he is a re-admissioner, the admitting department will usually only have the patient's name, address, telephone number, age, sex, diagnosis, and referring and attending doctors. The nursing unit usually has less information, the diagnostic and other departments often none. The resources of the hospital are then required for obtaining information which should be recorded elsewhere. For all elective admissions to hospital, a history, a description of pertinent findings, and a statement of the proposed diagnostic and treatment régime, should all be presented to the hospital prior to the admission of the patient. This should be, and hardly ever is, a mandatory condition of admission for the elective case.

Medical staff virtually never sets up criteria for admissions, for investigations and treatment, length of stay and discharge. Without the development of norms, hospital administration is severely handicapped in its efforts to ensure rational use of expensive in-patient facilities.

The private physician has been opposed to any significant change in the *status quo*, perhaps understandably, as Louis Lasagna suggested in a *New Republic* article: "... the practitioner of medicine is a member of the shrinking body of American entrepreneurs. Most doctors continue to 'run their own businesses' and are understandably opposed to interference in their economic affairs. . . ."

Yet, when discussing the direction and organization of our hospitals, it is vital to realize that the complexity of the medical care product demands an organized approach. It is no longer possible, in terms of either knowledge or cost for a single doctor to deliver a total medical product. Medical practice is inescapably an organizational process. However, this concept is difficult to accept even for society as a whole. It is double difficult for the entrepreneurial private physician to accept. John Kenneth Galbraith, the Harvard economist, describes the problem: "... to have, in pursuit of truth, to assert the superiority of the organization over the individual for important social tasks is a taxing prospect, yet it is a necessary task."

We are faced with the need for group action and positive control over the health environment. But who possesses this control now? Galbraith has made the observation: "On coming on any form of organized activity, a church, platoon, government, bureau, congressional committee, a house of casual pleasure, our first instinct is to inquire who is in charge. Then we inquire as to the qualifications or credentials which accord such command." In the hospital sector it is most difficult to determine who is actually in charge. There is a multiple set of answers. It is perhaps even more difficult to determine whether that individual or group of individuals, whoever he or they may be, are in fact qualified for command. However, in the majority of hospitals, control is exercised by the private physicians. It is this control, unresponsive to modern needs or public responsibility which is largely responsible for the shocking state of inefficiency and lowering of standards in North American hospitals.

Where to now? What hope exists? The problems of community hospitals that face North America at present will only be solved through recognition of our huge problem at all levels. Just building more hospitals and training more doctors is not the answer. Medical care must be looked on as an integrated system for advancing human needs. We must stop tackling the doctor, the hospital, financing, the delivery system, etc. as separate independent elements. They must be co-ordinated for the benefit of the society that created them. Decision-making in our community hospitals must begin to mean something. Bright administrators, not doctors, must run hospitals. Doctors must practice medicine. Incentives to improve care, reduce costs and improve efficiencies must be introduced at the national and community levels within individual facilities. We can no longer allow our hospitals to be doctors' workshops.

13
The Cost Spiral

One physician was paid $42,000 for administering 8,275 injections to 149 Medicare patients. – MEDICARE FINANCE COMMITTEE

In mid-winter 1970, I was talking with a legislative aide in Ottawa's Parliament Buildings and mentioned what seemed to me critical problems brought about by sky-rocketing costs in the medical and health care fields. Immediately the aide labelled me a backward-looking, *status quo* reactionary for discussing any aspect of costs in such an important area of social welfare. His attitude typifies that of many government officials in Washington and Ottawa. Too often they feel all that is needed to solve a problem is the passing of a law and the voting of massive sums of money.

Certainly governments must set goals in both social and welfare fields that will call for spending huge sums of tax dollars. Education, defense, transportation, health and medical programmes, the environment, our cities, all have legitimate claims on the public purse. Excessive waste in one area denies expenditures to other areas. What is worse, if expenditures are abnormally high in one particular area, this is a key indicator that the "guilty area" is plagued with waste and inefficiencies which seriously cripple its effectiveness. Such is the case with medical and health care services.

Many increases in costs have been justified and understandable but the majority have come about because of the waste, duplications and inefficiencies of the "non-system." Every chapter in this book in one way or another has touched upon subjects which affect costs.

By 1975, assuming present trends continue, North Americans will be spending approximately one hundred and ten billion dollars annually on health and medical care, which would be equivalent to about 8 per cent of the total gross national product of Canada and the United States.

In recent years, the United States has been spending more on medical care than on education or social security. Hospitals received 38 per cent or twenty-four billion of the total sixty-three billion 1970 outlay, doctors a 20 per cent slice, or twenty-four billion, drugs, 11 per cent, nursing homes 4 per cent, and hospital construction 4 per cent.

The 1970 sixty-three billion bill for health and medical services in the United States could easily reach two-hundred billion by the eighties. Some 40 per cent of the nation's bill is now paid by federal, state, and local governments. Commercial insurers pay 20 per cent and the people pay the rest.

Herman M. and Ann R. Somers in their book *Medicare And The Hospital* talk about the contemporary non-system being "the result of a haphazard growth of isolated, unco-ordinated institutions." Doctors are not cost conscious, and while some of the rise in costs is inevitable because of inflation, new medical technology and new life-saving developments, the real propellant forcing up costs is the archaic manner in which most medical care is arranged and paid for. "Almost nowhere else in the economy," says Victor R. Fuchs, a leading American economist "do technologists have as much control over demand." The only parallel, Fuchs says, is the military's control of the defense budget in time of total war.

Toward the end of 1970, the Economic Council of Canada reported, "Health care should be comprehensive and available to everyone as a matter of sound economic policy as well as on humane grounds." The Council cited duplication of services, loose co-ordination, limited long-range planning, and restrictive licensing practices by doctors as some of the main factors effecting the ever-increasing rise in costs. The Council found doctors' fees in Canada and the United States rising twice as fast as consumer prices, and hospital costs soaring five times faster. In Canada, in the period 1955 to 1968 health services costs nearly quadrupled from 1.2 billion to 4.4 billion dollars. Hospital care accounted for 55 per cent of the total increase. Expenditures have been increasing about 50 per cent faster than the gross national product, from $75.00 per capita in 1955 to $214.00 per capita in 1968. The increase for the same time period in the province was 700 per cent as the figure went from 271 million to 1.875 billion dollars. For municipalities during the same time, the figures doubled from 161 million to an estimated 335 million. The increase for the total expenditures of all three levels of government was six-fold from 535 million in 1955 to 3.075 billion in 1968. During the same period private expenditures doubled from an estimated 646 million to an estimated 1.370 billion. Canada's overall health bill is expected to reach a round figure of 14 billion dollars by 1980. The 1970 figure was 4.7 billion. Unless we act, the bill will have trebled in a decade.

Health care costs in Canada, already more than $200 each year for every man, woman and child, will soar to more than $550 per person by 1981, unless inefficiencies in the present system are eliminated and new methods introduced rapidly. We are currently faced with health care costs rising 10 per cent per year and hospital service costs rising 14 per cent annually.

In mid-1966, when Medicare and Medicaid went into effect in the United States, the price of medical care was already climbing twice as fast as the cost of living index. In 1950 the United States spent 11.1 billion for personal health service. By 1969, the same figure had reached 54.2 billion dollars.

Medicare is the main component of health expenditures to be financed by Washington and Ottawa. In our two countries, Medicare and Medicaid have been both the cause and the victims of sharply rising medical costs. During my first years as a member of parliament, it was heartbreaking to see lifetime savings depleted over night because of a sudden injury or illness. Since then, Ottawa and Washington have given more people access to services by voting income supplementation, but somewhere along the line they failed to extend existing services, or instigate essential new ones. As a result, they have subsequently put an intolerable load on an already overburdened health care system.

"Third-party" payment of medical bills through Blue Cross, Blue Shield and group insurance policies has provided another inflationary thrust. These companies have rarely scrutinized fees or the quality of services. Third-party laxity has most certainly increased the steep rise in hospital fees. As we have seen, cost controls are weak and sometimes non-existent in the hospital sector. While companies force patients into high-cost hospitals, the cost, plus reimbursement for services, is an open invitation to inefficiency.

Both in Canada and the United States the availability of money to pay bills under Medicare and Medicaid does not produce resources and services where they don't exist. As we have said, all over North America, in ghettos and rural areas, services are very limited, and sometimes nonexistent. A case in point is Pontiac County in Western Quebec where only four full-time doctors serve a population of 21,-000. As a result people often travel across the Ottawa River into Ontario when they need a doctor. They are understandably bitter about paying Quebec Medicare premiums without getting decent service. "If it wasn't for Ontario being located across the Ottawa River we wouldn't get any medical attention." says County Warden Basil Quaile. Medicare and Medicaid must be coupled with measures for imposing order on the distribution of services. Some authorities feel we are now wasting 40 per cent of the tax dollars we are pouring into the non-system. The North American taxpayer is not getting value for his health dollar.

What we choose to call Medicare and Medicaid in Canada and the United States is merely a finance mechanism designed by governments to help people pay for services in a system that these same governments consistently refuse to change in order to meet new conditions and soaring public demands. Governments pass out money, while showing no concern for the system and resources into which the money is put. By not preparing the system, the personnel and facilities to meet new expectations and demands, Ottawa and Washington have foisted a cruel and expensive hoax on the public. It is not the first time that centralized, "out of touch" authorities have put the cart before the horse by voting money for services that are not there. The shameful paradox is that the very low income people who are meant to be helped, are actually hurt while costs skyrocket.

For many doctors, Medicare and Medicaid have been a lucrative source of added income; for a few, the programmes have been a gold mine. Rashi Fein, Harvard Medical School professor of the economics of medicine, in 1969, told the Joint Congressional Economic Sub-Committee on Fiscal Policy: "After a bruising political battle to enact Medicare and Medicaid, government extended a hand of friendship to the medical community - and extended it in a most friendly way, by signing a blank cheque. The medical community was gracious and accepted the offer." Congress caved in under A.M.A. lobbying when passing Medicare and Medicaid. As a result, realistic financing plans were not implemented to bring about essential changes in the U.S. medical system.

The Finance Committee staff reported in 1969 that up to five thousand doctors had received payments of twenty-five thousand dollars or more from Medicare, and thousands of similar amounts from Medicaid.

Abuses cited by the Finance Committee included:

Gang visits, in which a physician might see as many as fifty patients in a day in one facility and charge each his full fee, regardless of whether the visits were medically necessary or whether a medical service was provided.

Unnecessary visits and unnecessary medical services were also cited. For example, one general practitioner billed Medicare in 1968 for $50,000 for house calls made to forty-nine patients. Another was paid

$42,000 for administering 8,275 injections to 149 Medicare patients, Fragmentary billing, in which a physician charges extra for services such as laboratory tests or psychiatric counseling that used to be included in routine charges for an office visit, were noted.

Payments to supervisory physicians in teaching hospitals were made for services where payments were not generally expected prior to Medicare. Conflict of interest, as a result of widespread physician investment in nursing homes and privately-owned hospitals, was also cited by the committee.

Canada is no better. The annual report of the Alberta Health Care Insurance Commission, tabled in the legislature, showed four doctors, all specialists, receiving payments of more than $240,000 each.

The average payment to the province's 1,418 doctors who earned over $10,000 was $43,430 with 42 pathologists averaging $124,508. Forty-nine doctors received payments of more than $100,000. General practitioners averaged $40,888. Specialists averaged $52,292, but the average for pathologists and radiologists was $108,593.

The majority of North American physicians are operating on their own, as private entrepreneurs. They have become an army of push-cart vendors in an age of supermarkets; meanwhile, they are in the leading income brackets in both countries. Physicians' average incomes in Canada in 1946 were $7,466 and in 1966, $24,993 – a 300 per cent rise in two decades. A recent edition of *Fortune* magazine pointed out, "Most patients pay a piecework method of fees for service, with separate billings for visits to the doctor, shots, X-Rays, lab tests, surgery, anesthesia, hospital room and board."

Prepaid group-practice plans could go a long way in reducing costs, yet in the United States organized medicine, led by the American Medical Association, continues to lobby and oppose such obviously efficient changes. In seventeen states, laws still prohibit the ownership and operation of group practices by consumer-oriented groups.

In 1963 the Sault Ste. Marie, Ontario Group Health Centre opened its doors, amid controversy and discord with the local medical profession. A lay, non-profit corporation, it was sponsored by a local of the Steelworkers' Union and community representatives. It built, and now operates, a medical facility for group medical practice. The facility has gained wide recognition as a high-quality medical care institution, in which modern group practice of medicine is combined with prepayment of the costs of care along with consumer participation in the provision of health care facilities. But it has received little acclaim in medical circles.

The near-breakdown, financially, of the North American non-system can, in part, be laid at Washington's and Ottawa's doorstep. Dr. James A. Shannon, criticizes both the twenty-four federal agencies and the bureau of the budget for failing to present a satisfactory analysis of health spending in the 1970 budget. In particular he stressed the absence of the aggregate "Federal Health Dollar" that had "real relationship to the civilian needs of the nation." As a result, Dr. Shannon said, "The nation lacked a clear understanding of the federal commitment to health, and the congress was not presented with an intellectually honest analysis of federal funds that will be expended for the health maintenance of the population."

Shannon continued, "In the longer view, federal resources should be used to influence the operation of systems that are essential for the ultimate satisfaction of the health needs of all the people. Within this view, the federal government has identified research, education, and the provision of facilities as primary responsibilities to be shared in varying degrees with the non-federal sectors. Few even general goals are established and major health deficiencies are not defined. The system is in danger of catastrophic breakdown. Health activities are distributed ubiquitously within the executive agencies, lacking either central policy direction or broad programme goals as a base for programme development. In effect, the budget analysis document clearly portrays an unsatisfactory frame of reference for an essential and important federal function."

If the intention is really to move a sluggish system in a new direction, then funds for new construction are woefully inadequate in Canada and the United States. Both federal governments have asserted their broad and direct responsibility with regard to the maintenance of the health of the population, but they ignore their commitment to help solve the problems of the system.

North American federal outlays support a combination of programmes that should provide the knowledge necessary for managing the problems of health maintenance and fighting disease; provide for the development of systems of health care that are directed toward satisfying the needs of major segments of the population; and produce an adequate health manpower pool and the essential physical facilities.

To begin doing this, intelligent management is needed. Ottawa's

Public Accounts Committee, which examines government expenditures, and the Auditor General's office, which does the same job, both agree that health and medical care expenditures top the list for waste and lack of central controls. Internal auditing within Canada's Department of National Health and Welfare, unlike most departments, is virtually non-existent.

Looking, in more detail, into the North American scene, hospital costs, alone, bear specific review. Hospital patient day costs rose by an annual average of 7.5 per cent over the past decade in the United States. In Canada, hospital costs amount to two billion annually and, as we said, are now increasing at an annual rate of 14 per cent. American Hospital Association representatives recently testified before the House Ways and Means Committee that the average daily room rate would rise to nearly $100 a day by 1973. From 1946 to 1969 hospital daily service charges in the United States increased 592 per cent, almost seven times as fast as all prices, and almost five times as fast as all services in the Consumer Price Index.

In one Toronto hospital, bed costs doubled in five years. Today a bed in the hospital costs as much as $85.78 per day. The same bed in 1965 cost $41.56 per day.

The Royal Victoria Hospital in Montreal is typical of North American community hospitals. In 1963, the hospital had twenty-four thousand two hundred and eight admissions and total expenditures of $13,692,283. By 1969, admission were down to twenty thousand and forty-three while total expenditures rose to $25,849,767.

Until the end of the thirties, physicians' services accounted for the largest single share of the United States health dollar. By 1940, hospitals had moved in front and have increased their share steadily since. Between 1940 and 1968, hospital costs moved from 26 per cent to 36 per cent of the health dollar.

Certainly there is justification for some hospital cost increases, and some of those most frequently advanced are medical and hospital technology which have advanced at a phenomenal pace, with commensurate demands on facilities, equipment, personnel, and services. Those admitted use more services per capita, such as diagnostic and therapeutic X-Ray procedures, drugs, and laboratory services. There has also been a growth in the range of services made available. For example, between 1963 and 1968, the proportion of community hospitals with intensive care services (including coronary care services) jumped from 18 per cent to 42 per cent. The equipment for all such

107

services grows more elaborate and costly, and its rate of obsolescence more rapid. There are two other major factors involved in rising costs. First, there has been a trend away from acute but brief illness; instead, hospitals are receiving patients with expensive, long-term ailments. Second, hospitals have finally begun to pay better salaries, while at the same time improving working conditions and reducing the hours of work. This costs money and, I might point out again, has been long overdue.

Increased payroll costs are the major factor in hospital operating costs. But it is not true that payroll costs have advanced more rapidly than other costs in recent years. From 1960 to 1968, despite a substantial rise in personnel in relation to patient load, total expenses per patient day advanced more rapidly than payroll per patient day: 90 per cent against 82 per cent. Payrolls accounted for 62 per cent of total expenses in 1960 and 60 per cent in 1968.

Moreover, wage increases cannot be charged with the whole responsibility for payroll increases. The American Hospital Association attributes half of increased total expenditures for wages and salaries between 1963 and 1968 to additional employment. The hospitals are accused of an insatiable capacity for absorbing more manpower, the only restraint being their availability. They had an alleged manpower crisis in 1950, when hospitals were employing 178 persons per 100 in-patients; now there are 272 employees per 100 in-patients, a striking increase of 53 per cent which cannot be fully explained by the growth of services.

Hospitals have assumed increased functions in addition to direct patient care. Important among these is education. Despite the decline in hospital-based schools of nursing, they still account for about four-fifths of registered nurse graduates, and the cost of these programmes to the hospitals is rising. With federal subsidies for nurse education and the trend toward academic settings for such education, this burden should eventually decline, but it will do so slowly. Also, many hospitals have been adding full-time directors of medical education, an additional, although modest, factor in costs.

Critics of hospital costs do not find such explanations satisfying. As statements of fact, they are true, as far as they go. Certainly it cannot be questioned that there has been a great expansion of facilities, equipment, personnel, and services. But how much represents unnecessary duplication of facilities and equipment among several hospitals within the same community, because each hospital behaves

108

as an autonomous unit, rather than as part of a coordinated health care system? How much of the new equipment is merely for prestige or convenience?

How much of the mounting increase in ancilliary services is simply a result of the spread of third-party payment, which has reduced the physicians' reluctance to allow additional laboratory precedures or an additional day's stay in hospital, and the individual consumer's resistance to higher costs, on which a normal market situation would place considerable reliance?

Has there been any attempt to measure the relative value to health care represented by new equipment and added services, or are "improved models" bought because hospitals now have a virtual guarantee of repayment of all their costs from third-party payors? Has there been progress toward developing measures of cost-benefit relationships?

Another reason for rising costs is, of course, drugs. Any grassroots politician who has kept in touch with his people is continuously faced with the pleas, especially of older people, in this regard. Far too often I witnessed elderly couples attempting to survive on a little over $200 a month and spending up to $50 per month on drugs.

Generally, the price charged for a prescription includes the cost of the drug supplied and the pharmacist's dispensing fee. Time and time again, doctors write prescriptions which people just plainly cannot afford and they are not filled out. Some companies in fact give selected products to hospitals and count on recovering the loss through retail sales. The patient out of the hospital actually subsidizes the patient in the hospital.

Doctors should be persuaded to prescribe a limited number of prescriptions, using generic, rather than brand names. One brand of tranquilizers in Montreal retails for $12.00 for a bottle of one hundred pills. An identical product, sold under the generic name, sells for $4.00 per hundred. The Winnipeg businessman who needed the tranquilizer, stelazine, could pay as high as $15.50 per hundred, compared to his Montreal colleague who could get the same quantity for $7.60. A Vancouver housewife could obtain the contraceptive ortho-novum for $1.69 per twenty pills, at the cheapest, while the housewives of Halifax might have to pay as high as $2.50 for the same number.

This spread between the highest and lowest prices for common prescribed drugs was found in nineteen drugs checked by the Department of Consumer and Corporate Affairs officials in the retail drugstores of five Canadian cities in May 1970.

Other examples of the spread were:

The tranquilizer, librium, which could be purchased at the lowest price in Vancouver for $4.69 per hundred; the highest price found was $10.85 per hundred tablets in Montreal.

The hormone pill, premarin, which could be obtained most cheaply in Winnipeg at $6.94 per hundred, reached a high of $11.50 per hundred in Halifax.

The antibiotic, tetrex, was selling for as low as $3.34 and as high as $9.00, for twenty-five capsules, in Montreal.

The stimulant, pulverized tuinal, was available at $2.39 in Montreal, but could cost as high as $5.60 in Vancouver, at least $1.60 above all other cities tested.

Individual pharmacists who attempt to lower prices can count on little support from their protective associations or colleagues. Morrie Neiss, owner of a drug store in Montreal, found this out early in January, 1971. The Quebec College of Pharmacists ostensibly wanted his licence suspended for the official reason that he was selling soap flakes and dogs' leashes.

Jean Décarie was president of the Quebec College of Pharmacists from 1963 to 1966. He attempted to devise a means of making low-cost prescriptions available, especially in poorer areas of Montreal. The College governors could not agree on how this could be done. On relinquishing the presidency, Décarie set about attempting to show it *could* be done, and has been hounded by College inspectors ever since.

In 1967, the House of Commons Committee on Drug Costs and Prices pointed the finger at pharmacists as being a major factor in high-cost drugs. Four years later the situation has worsened. In Quebec, one out of four prescriptions is never filled because the recipient cannot afford the charge.

The United States and Canada have similar drug marketing systems. They are among the most restrictive in the world. Drug prices in Canada and the United States are substantially higher than in other countries. Leading United States firms avoid price competition. A recent *Wall Street Journal* report cites a memorandum of the United States Anti-Trust Division as follows: "Our investigation indicates certain pharmaceutical manufacturers sought to restrict, control and monopolize United States foreign commerce in pharmaceutical products, particularly prescription drugs. It also reveals that such companies have combined and conspired among themselves and with others to restrain both United States imports and exports of these products and to foreclose foreign markets to United States' competitors."

In Canada, the big drug manufacturers spend millions on sales promotion to "sell" doctors their brand-name drugs; the doctor prescribes these expensive brand-names because he has confidence in them, and because he is probably not familiar with their generic equivalents or alternatives; the pharmacist, with his dispensing monopoly, fills the prescription at a profit that seldom bears much relationship to the professional service performed.

The system of retail distribution of drugs in North America resembles "a cartel . . . or a guild from the Middle Ages," according to a report on drug distribution for the Quebec Commission on Health. It states that no comprehensive public health service can properly be developed until pharmacists abandon outdated professional practices and regulations, and adds, "The economic universe of professionalism is that of a corporation of artisans which tries to reduce to a minimum every external pressure towards efficiency, dynamism, and the need to reduce costs."

Drugs are only one facet in health care, but it is obvious from their high price, and from the other conditions we have touched on in this chapter, that adequate care for all North Americans is impossible unless all the costs are brought under control.

The provisions of health care is a classic economic problem. Human and non-human care resources are scarce. Thus it is necessary to choose which of many health goods and services to produce and, as an added complication, there generally are alternative ways of combining one or more scarce health care resources to provide particular health goods. The scarcity of health care resources reflects the general scarcity of resources in the economy at large, all the more reason why good sense, cost control, and humane management techniques should prevail. All the more reason governments should effect and impress the system the people are paying for with their own tax dollars.

It is right that our energies are now engaged in the paramount and immediate struggle to employ more effectively and equitably the great resources we invest in health services. But we must remember that health services do not alone bring health. Even if we attain full equality in services for the poor, their health status will remain unequal. Health services will not overcome the disadvantages of poverty itself, the consequences of inferior housing, food, recreation, and education. For other groups as well, as the level of health services rises, a point of diminishing returns from such services may be reached, as compared with investment in the quality of the living environment. Thus we may have to decide between making minimal improvements in health care or meeting other social needs. The time for such frankly acknowledged choices may not be very far away.

14
Health Maintenance and Preventive Medicine

The health of the people is really the foundation upon which all their happiness and all their powers as a state depend – BENJAMIN DISRAELI

It is often difficult to draw a distinct line between preventive medicine and active cure treatment for patients already suffering from disease, sickness or injury. This should, hopefully, become more difficult in the future, when medical care involves the total medical and health care requirements of individual citizens. One thing we do know is that what health maintenance defines as "not sick" does not necessarily imply genuine good health.

Too many of us go to the doctor when it is too late. Regular check-ups could prevent a great deal of pain and suffering. Yet is this entirely the fault of the public? We tend to think of the doctor and his helpers as terribly over-worked and feel a little sheepish about taking his time for an examination when we are feeling fit. This should not be so. So much of our medical and health care effort is directed toward putting out "bush fires" and chasing horses that have already escaped through unlocked doors. We are much more likely to take precautions against fire than precautions to prevent disease, injury and sickness.

In a supposedly free society we are reluctant to develop or implement effective programmes of public health education. This is especially true if such programmes turn out to be in conflict with vested interests. Public health doctors are bad at trying to communicate knowledge and information to the public. There is a terrible and scandalous gap between knowledge and its application. A large part of what the public hears about health is based on the deliberate attempt to activate fear, and people refuse to listen. Fear should be forgotten and self-interest should be cmphasized. Meaningful, regular physical examinations should be encouraged. Well-women's clinics, where the cancer pap smear test is performed, should involve more and more women. Millions of women still don't get this test for detecting cancer of the cervix.

113

Why do over forty thousand people die annually in North America because of colon and rectal cancer, when simple proctological examination, if done in time, according to the American Cancer Society, could save close to thirty thousand of these lives? Poor or non-existent communications underlie the problem. Our medical schools do a disgraceful job at teaching preventive techniques, while the hospital sector is almost totally directed toward active treatment. Individual doctors and hospitals play little, and often no, part in the community responsibility of preventive medicine.

We treat tuberculosis patients when we should be treating the air they breathe. We allow hospital incinerators to spew waste into the atmosphere. We attempt to cure diseases and allow open garbage dumps to dot the North American map from coast to coast. How often do we ask the following questions: How can a community know when it is harbouring the centre of a disease? How can it prevent the outbreak of that disease? What is the community doing to prevent the introduction of disease? What are the effects of man's alteration of his own environment? Does changing the normal ecology of the community also change the mechanisms of disease transmission?

In talking about prevention, some groups underline the importance of consumer protection and adequate safeguards in the production and distribution of foods, drugs, alcohol, and devices intended for the use of the ultimate consumer. Others emphasize attacks on major diseases by health experts and related agencies. They point to the success of immunizing agents and their proven effectiveness to shield the consumer from tetanus, polio, diptheria, whooping cough and measles.

In North America, in the last half-century, we have noted the defeat of one vicious disease after another: Yellow fever, malaria, smallpox, cholera. In 1952, there were over sixty thousand cases of polio in Canada and the United States. By 1969, in both countries, there were less than one hundred and fifty. Yet, in spite of the high degree of protection enjoyed by North Americans, death comes annually to over one hundred and fifty thousand people as a result of communicable diseases.

Unconquered diseases fall into two major categories. Those for which we have adequate control measures which are not being used to the fullest extent and, secondly, those for which control measures do not exist and for which they are not adequate. For polio, diptheria, whooping cough and tetanus, we have safe and effective vaccines.

Yet, when the *Vaccination Assistance Act* was passed in the United States in 1962, eleven million children under five were not protected against these diseases.

In 1965 nearly four and a half million North American children caught measles, which can cause mental retardation. For many other diseases, there are no control measures whatsoever. We are still looking for effective vaccines against german measles, hepatitis, encephalitis, and the common cold. We have influenza vaccines available, but the viruses are constantly changing their character.

Many modern phenomena have both a direct and indirect effect on general preventive measures. Automation is a case in point, as it often means minimal physical demands. The loss of recreational facilities, as a result of building developments, freeways, parking lots, and other products of urbanization does not enhance health and physical fitness. Many of us get the car out of the garage to drive for three minutes to the corner drug store. René Duclos once said, "Who can foretell the distant consequences of the fact that modern man no longer experiences the inclemencies of the weather, need not engage in physical exertion, can use drugs to alleviate almost any form of pain, and increasingly depends upon tranquilizers and stimulants to live through the day? These achievements have, of course, made life easier and often more pleasant, but they may bring about an atrophy of the adoptive mechanisms which continue to be essential for the maintenance of health."

The Importance of Exercise

Automation and the everyday habits of modern man leads us directly to physical fitness as yet another consideration in the field of prevention. How often have we heard, "I haven't got time to exercise." Physical training must be worked at regularly. Whether we like it or not, the body begins to deteriorate after the age of 26. From that time forward we become subject to the sagging abdomen, the hernia, hemorrhoids, and varicose veins. Vascular diseases increase and the heart and brain become more vulnerable. Atrophy and deterioration progress more slowly when we are physically fit. We reduce stress, anxiety, insomnia and possibly emotional breakdown. Yet, there are far too many North American spectators, and far too many golf carts. We need exercise programmes that last after school and college years. We allow ourselves to deteriorate too early. We must adjust our working day to find time for proper exercise, suited to each individual situation. Maybe people live longer now than ever before in history. Nevertheless, we lose our effectiveness much too soon.

What's Wrong With What We Eat and Drink

Today many authorities stress the importance of diet, nutrition and exercise. More particularly, they have an obvious application in the field of prevention. Cardiovascular diseases are surely a case in point. Here we deal with such things as total caloric need, exercise, the prevention of obesity, the relative amounts of different fats in the diet and the cholesterol content of the diet. Proper nutrition, say some experts, could lessen the early incidence of coronary heart disease by 20 per cent. The spectacle of the sagging, over-sized North American living in an automated urbanized society and consuming too many calories in over-processed or synthetic foods, speaks for itself. North America holds the unenviable record for the world's highest mortality rate from uncontrolled heart disease.

Let's just look at the way we eat for a few minutes. For the past number of decades the quality of the North American diet has been allowed to deteriorate criminally. Citizens of Canada and the United States eat poorly, no matter how affluent we believe our society to be. The effect of this poor diet on our national health picture cannot be overstated. North America's largest retail industry has been allowed to let the safety, wholesomeness and value of their products decline shamefully. The Food and Drug Administrations, on both sides of the border have, so far, failed in their missions.

It has always been a standard joke that each of us consumes a few bushels of dirt in our lifetime. This was serious enough in the years when populations were relatively near to a natural food supply. It is doubly serious, now, in our increasingly urbanized society because, in the name of processing and preserving, our food is coloured, treated, added to, and affected by pesticides and other chemicals. The results are grave.

As is obvious, food plays a wide role in the field of preventative medicine. Not only because we don't eat what we should, but also because we too frequently eat (and drink) what we shouldn't. We'll pass over the too-well documented cases of mercury poisoning, but it would be well to recall here the strange case of the Quebec beer drinkers heart-disease epidemic.

In October, 1967, the Canadian Medical Association revealed that cobalt sulphate, a chemical added to beer to maintain the picturesque foam on top, had been found responsible for the death of twenty Quebec City beer drinkers. The detailed investigation carried out by twenty-one medical investigators, and led by Dr. Y. L. Morin, Director of the Institute of Cardiology at Laval University, proved that cobalt sulphate played a significant role in the sudden appearance of forty-eight cases of acute heart failure, due to alcoholic cardiomyopathy (a heart disease) and the twenty deaths that occurred in Quebec City between August, 1965 and March, 1966. The facts, as described below, are all taken directly from material gathered by Dr. Morin and his team of investigators.

The forty-eight people, two of whom were women, ranged in ages from 25 to 66. They were all heavy beer drinkers and had been for a long time. The majority of them drank over 200 ounces of beer per day – a few as much as 500 ounces. The report stated, "It is apparent that the length of time the person had been a heavy drinker was more important than the amount he drank per day."

One brand of beer, Dow Ale, produced by Canadian Breweries, Canada's largest brewing company and credited with having 80 per cent of the Quebec City beer market, was blamed for the epidemic. "The disease appeared one month after the Dow brand was made with the additive (cobalt sulphate) and no further cases were seen a month after the chemical had been removed."

There were no other cases detected in other areas, in spite of a thorough search by medical authorities. Dow Ale had also been produced in Montreal, yet no cases were discovered there. The report added that the concentration of cobalt in the Quebec City beer (1.2 parts per million) was much higher than in the Montreal product (0.075 p.p.m.) and that in Montreal, only draft beer contained cobalt, while in Quebec City both draft and bottled beer contained the higher concentration of cobalt. The combination produced a much higher intake of cobalt in the Quebec City beer drinkers.

A similar epidemic, involving sixty-four cases had been underway in Omaha, Nebraska, for a full year prior to the Quebec experience. When cobalt was discovered to be the cause in Quebec, Omaha authorities were notified. The cobalt was removed from the Omaha beer and after one month no additional cases were discovered. The blame in the case may be obscure to some, yet here are some further facts. Dr. Morin stated, "There is an antidote for cobalt poisoning in animals. It might have saved some of our patients had we known the metal to be present in beer at the time." Yet, investigators were unable to obtain from government authorities or the brewing industry the cobalt content of beers, even though there was conclusive proof that an additive precipitated the death of twenty Canadians.

Even as late as 1971, medical investigators and publicly-elected representatives to parliament were still unable to obtain from government authorities or industry either a description of the additives and chemicals going into foods and beverages, or a statement of the quantities used.

The Quebec City case is an outstanding example of inadequate health measures taken to protect the consumers. The story of cyclamates in our diet-crazy society is another.

In the United States, the first association of the F.D.A. with a cyclamate product came in January 1950 when Abbott Laboratories filed a new drug application for sucaryl. F.D.A. tests showed the appearance of malignant tumors in animals. Still, Washington ruled that sucaryl could go on the market. On August 10, 1959, three years and nine months after, the food committee of the National Academy of Sciences recommended against "the uncontrolled distribution of foodstuffs containing cyclamates." F.D.A. declared in relation to non-nutritive sweetners "safety has been adequately established for the substance in this category." Soon nearly 75 per cent of families in the United States would be consuming cyclamates. By 1966, two Japanese scientists reported that cyclamates passing through the body of a man could create a different chemical called cyclohexiglamine (C.H.A.). Later tests showed this occurred in about one-third of the population. C.H.A. is clearly a dangerous drug. Yet, the Directorates in Canada and the United States ignored one danger signal after another. When Secretary Finch finally removed cyclamates from the Generally Recognized As Safe (G.R.A.S.) list, he did not mention the doubts which had been in evidence throughout fifteen years of research regarding this chemical, which should never have been allowed on the market.

In 1969, North American food industry sales amounted to over one hundred and twenty-five billion dollars. Economically, the North American industry is moving by merger to monopoly and most of the recent growth in the food industry is in processed foods, such as pre-cooked breakfast cereals, with all the food value taken out of them.

The Food and Drug Directorates on both sides of the border are simply not equipped to meet the new challenge. Treating the chemicals in these cereals, with their genetic and birth-defect potential, as casually as they treated cyclamates ten years ago, Ottawa and Washington, are sowing the seeds of disaster for the 1980's. But they have been clearly warned.

Foods high in starch, salt and sugar are replacing the fruits, vegetables, or meats of twenty years ago. Further to this, in both Canada and the United States, 70 per cent of all food standards are initially proposed by the food industry itself. Procedures in Ottawa and Washington, deciding what chemicals are safe, have so distorted the laws that nothing practical has been left of their provisions. Even though our problems are multiplying in geometric proportions, neither government has exerted any control over the rapidly developing food market since 1968. Fewer than half of the twenty-five hundred food additives in use in North America have been tested, and it is expected the number of food additives will have approximately doubled by 1974.

F.D.A. food standards and exemptions now in force in the United States and Canada read like a catalogue of favours to special interests. Hundreds of conferences between F.D.A. officials and industry representatives take place every month. Rarely in the "democratic" society is the consumer so poorly represented. The resulting damage cannot be measured. One thing we do know, most North Americans, because of poor nutrition and adulterated food have been deprived of many of the benefits which we could normally have expected from advances in medical and health science.

What About "The Pill"?

The government is supposed to be our watchdog in the field of health and drugs. Yet what good is a watchdog that only watches? Consider, for instance, the case of "The Pill." When the pill for women was put on the North American market, original claims and guarantees gave no cause for concern regarding side effects. But, now we realize it was over nine years after the original marketing of this birth control drug before any meaningful testing was initiated by the National Institute of Health in Washington. Today it is clearly evident that the pill should only be taken after full examination by a doctor, and those taking it should have regular check-ups. What has been learned about the pill? An investigation started by Doctor B. Herzley and Doctor

Alex Cappen at the Medical Research Council's Neurosphyschiatric Unit in Carshalton, England, found that one in ten women taking oral contraceptives was subject to severe depression. Some investigations have noted a marked increase in the suicide rate from women on the pill.

Doctor Helen Taussig, Professor Emeritus of Pediatrics at Johns Hopkins Hospital, Baltimore, Maryland, has pointed to the risk from the pill for women with weak hearts. She claims "Giving the pill to these women has produced more fatal results than we like to see." United States' Brain Surgeon, Doctor Clark Milliken of the University of Minnesota, links the pill with some strokes. "The pill," he said, "should not be taken by any woman who has had a fleeting interruption of blood supply to the brain, often called a small stroke." Doctor Charles Scott of the University of Utah, claims the pill may cause chromosome damage and birth defects.

It seems only too obvious that the original testing on the pill left much to be desired. Still the Food and Drug administration in the United States will not make public administration records on clinical testing of oral contraceptives, and on June 30, 1970, Mrs. Carolyn D. M. Morgan filed a lawsuit in United States District Court, Washington, for access to Food and Drug's records on clinical tests of the pill.

The controversy still rages. Doctor Paul Brazeau, a Quebec biologist at the University of Sherbrooke, warns that teenagers, who go on the pill before they are sexually mature, may be stunted in growth.

One of the leading cases involving "the pill" was brought up by a Brooklyn widow, Mrs. Roberta Meinert. Mrs. Meinert sued on the grounds that she received intestinal damage from the drug, and was awarded $251,000. She used the pill "Enovid" in 1961 and 1962, which was produced by the Chicago-based company G.D. Searle, and soon found herself suffering from phlebitis, a blood-clotting disease. Mrs. Meinert incurred a severe thrombosis in her intestines before having parts of her intestines removed during two operations. Counsel for the widow – stated Searle – knew of cases of death caused from the pill after blood-clotting.

Why Do We Legalize Smoking?

Many leading authorities feel there are well over three hundred thousand premature deaths in North America each year because of the nicotine habit. Incredible as it may sound, the American Medical Association accepted ten million dollars for research from the tobacco companies. Consequently, it came as no surprise when the A.M.A. refused to endorse United States Surgeon General Terry's report on smoking and health. Heavy smoking can cut several years off your life, to say nothing about reducing your effectiveness and pleasure.

Can We Save Our Environment?

In recent years, perhaps no subject relating to the concept of prevention has received more attention than the environment. Unfortunately, this has resulted, to date, in minimal action. As Ralph Nader stated in Montreal in April of 1970, "We've had a pretty heavy dose of pollution for twenty years now, and the effects are becoming evident." Nader described pollution as "a massive form of environmental violence inflicted against the will of the individual."

Winston Churchill once wrote, "We shape our buildings and afterwards our buildings shape us." René Duclos, in his inaugural address for the opening of the Pan-American Health Building in Washington, said "Medically speaking, man is more the product of his environment than of his genetic endowment. The most important health problems in the world today have their origins in man's total response to his total environment."

Canada and the United States have seen a massive deterioration of environmental quality in our overcrowded cities. Our countryside suffers from exploitation, litter, blight and industrial dereliction. We use streams as sewers and pollute our water, our soil and our air. We have wonder drugs and spotless operating theatres, but they are, at best, cures and not preventatives. What are some of the results of this situation?

Dr. Ernest Mastromatteo, director of the Ontario Department of Health's environmental health services said, "Pollution may be the reason that the life expectancy of middle-aged men has decreased slightly in recent years. The Dominion Bureau of Statistics has reported that a fifty-five year old Canadian man can expect to live 75.3 years, but a forty-five year old man can expect to live only 73.4 years."

The North American environment frequently breeds allergies. Dr. A. H. Eisen, head of Montreal's Children's Hospital's allergy and clinical immunology department says that North American life tends to encourage the development of allergies and possibly asthmatic conditions. He noted, for instance, that immigrant families who come from all parts of the world complain of allergies they never had in their own countries. Tragically, there is strong evidence that our bad air hits our children very hard. Dr. David Bates, an internationally recognized expert on the health effects of air pollution, said that air pollution in Canada's major cities is striking deep into the lungs of the youngest children and boosting their chances of serious chest troubles in later life.

Bates, the chairman of physiology at Montreal's McGill University, based his claim on two studies of children and air pollution, one involving four thousand infants in the United Kingdom and another with several hundred infants in Montreal. The six-year United Kingdom study found that infections in the lower respiratory system were four times more common in children raised in high-pollution areas compared to low pollution areas. Considered a classic piece of research, the United Kingdom study avoided the pitfall of genetic patterns among the subjects, by focusing on four thousand children adopted at birth.

Current pollution readings in large Canadian cities, Montreal, Toronto, Vancouver, indicated that children under two years of age are suffering an increased burden of diseases because of air pollution. A 50 per cent pollution cut would probably add five years to babies' lives. Deaths from lung cancer and, in fact, all lung disease, would be cut by 25 per cent. All disease and death would be reduced by a 4.5 per cent yearly average, with an annual saving to the Canadian nation of at least two billion dollars.

The following evaluations of the human price of dirty air, based on existing medical knowledge, were made by two Pittsburgh economists, Lester Lave and Eugene Seskin of the Carnegie-Mellen School of Industrial Administration, and were presented before a pollution symposium in Washington in 1970.

The economists found that merely easing pollution in acute periods, like those that have hit cities in summer, would have little effect on overall death and disease rates. It is the lesser but constant pollution that is important, they concluded, not the occasional peaks. People dealing with this problem should worry about abating air pollution at all times, instead of confining their concern to increased pollution during inversions.

The effect of air pollution on lung cancer and bronchial ailments are striking, and second only to the effects of cigarette smoking.

In summary, the effects are strong in the deaths of both the old and the very young. There are strong correlations between deaths of infants up to eleven months old with atmospheric concentrations of sulphuric acid and dust. Lave believes, "For the middle-class American family living in an urban area, abating air pollution is the single most important thing we could do to improve health. If we could reduce air pollution by fifty per cent, it would save nearly as much in money and life as if we found a complete cure for cancer."

When thinking about the air left to breathe, we should recognize that 95 per cent of the total air supply exists in the layer extending only twelve miles above the surface of the earth. In North America, the level of air pollution is rapidly increasing. More than eighty million motor vehicles discharge about three hundred thousand tons of nitrogen oxides every day. Approximately one hundred and ten thousand tons of sulphur and sulphur oxide from the burning of sulphur containing coal and petroleum products such as fuel oil in homes, power plants and industries, are added to our air each day. We cannot yet, completely, measure air pollution effects on health because so much of it is recent. Yet nearly all authorities agree the effects are most serious and little is being done. When there is doubt, it is rarely resolved in favour of health and, with air pollution, there is no way to capture the pollutants in the community atmosphere once they have been released.

A further immediate priority includes the development of a comprehensive water programme for all North America. In 1886, the Massachusetts Legislature passed an act to protect the purity of the inland waters. The initial objective was the control of water-borne disease. Today's urbanization, population growth, stepped up agricultural production and resource development, are accompanied by major increases in the synthesis and manufacture of chemicals and their resultant pollution of the atmosphere and hydrosphere. The cry now is for an adequate supply of clean water. In North America, over 30 per cent of all cities have an inadequate public water supply. In our age of scientific sophistication, we still fluoridate the water supply of only a quarter of the people in North America. In North America, twenty-eight million septic tanks are still discharging into roadside ditches and the streets, spewing sewage into backyards and neighbouring wells.

In the development of a comprehensive water programme, government institutions will have to adapt and change radically. This is a

123

challenge that knows no borders. The pollution of the Great Lakes is just one example. There is no agreement about tackling the problem, and the result is next to no action, while we transform the world's largest inland waters into cesspools. The institutional machinery for dealing with them should be consigned to a constitutional museum. It involves and requires agreement between Ottawa, Washington, the states and provinces, counties, cities and towns surrounding the lakes and the International Joint Commission. Needless to say, the necessary agreement has not been forthcoming as our once-magnificent lakes die before our eyes.

What are some of the immediate changes we must look for in North American environmental health? Specifically, we must envisage more planning and zoning in urban and rural areas, and the modification and probable elimination of the internal combustion engine. Burning combustibles can and should often be replaced with nuclear and hydro-electric power. Vast changes in our transportation systems are also involved.

We know what we mean when we talk about private and public property. My house is my private property. The local post office is public property. But what about the air above, our shorelines, lakes and rivers? It would be correct to call them "unrestricted common property." Everybody uses them, but nobody has the obligation of conserving them in a decent state. Our air, water and soil often fall into the category of "unrestricted common property," as they steadily deteriorate. Positive legal developments must deal with this pressing emergency, for land in medieval times was exploited to nothing when there were no vested property rights.

Both Washington and Ottawa must establish anti-pollution ground rules. We cannot always blame industry when there are no rules. I am convinced if government would only act, modern technology, coupled with the conscience of the vast majority of responsible contemporary business leaders, would meet the challenge.

The whole question of environmental health impinges on a host of factors in the area of prevention. When thinking of air, soil, water and noise pollution, we should be more positive and also consider the greater advantages contained in planning for better living space, a more effective use of the earth's surface, regional planning, housing, occupational health, esthetics and beauty. Pollution must be stopped at the source.

In cleaning up our environment, negative attitudes can have no place. The whole challenge must be met in a positive frame of mind by both the public and government. Modern planning and modern technology will and should take account of beauty, excellence, non-obsolescence and quality. Basing our approach on these ideas will be a greater spur to action in a field which directly involves health maintenance and the prevention of disease.

Mental Health – What We Need to Achieve It

A systematic approach to environmental health is imperative. We need not just the technical answers to existing problems, but a better comprehension of what the larger problems and larger issues really are and how they should be approached. We need to conserve and utilize natural resources in such a way as to prevent disease and to assure an environment in conformity with the highest aspirations of the human spirit. Many of the effects of man on his environment and environment on man are both predictable and preventable. Questions of mental health and the problems created by our urban world are demanding more and more attention. Poverty, over-crowding, transportation, discrimination – all are considerations, all effect the whole man, and wholeness must be the goal of sound mental health. The preventative aspect of mental health is, perhaps, the most complex of all preventative problems. Yet one thing is certain. We must start attacking the social causes of mental illness. If not, we shall continue to tackle the all-but-endless task of caring for its recurring effects. Alcoholism, drug addiction, juvenile delinquency – all, in part, relate to the environment.

Housing conditions are but one example of effects on mental health and skills. It was reported in England in 1970 at a meeting of the British Association for the Advancement of Science, from a survey of sixteen thousand school children: "We find that when allowance is made for all other factors, seven-year-old children, living in over-crowded homes, are retarded by nine months in reading age." In Canada, we have, by any definition, over five hundred thousand sub-standard dwellings affecting over three million Canadians.

Basic to the maintenance of mental health is the recognition that a person is more likely to avoid mental disorder if he learns how to handle himself effectively in unexpected stress situations. Premature submission to, or evasion of, problems is a danger which often leads to mental disorder, flights into magical thinking, fantasy, alienation or the development of other neurotic symptoms. From these experiences we arrive at some notion of preventative psychiatry, embodying the idea of helping people to increase their ability to solve unexpected problems. Such a goal can only be achieved by enlightened education, and by finding ways of assisting people when they are struggling with a current life crisis. Exposure to stress and challenge gives us a higher tolerance for ambiguity and frustration.

All over North America we need more comprehensive community mental health centres and public health psychiatry. Psychiatrists offer invaluable specific services, but they must move beyond this and incorporate their findings regarding the needs of human development into the process of social planning and change. Social and welfare services lack co-ordination, and frequently treat the individual as if he were not one, but twenty different people. To find methods of improving mental health would mean fewer psychiatric breakdowns, and this is a vital aim, since the mental health of North Americans cannot depend upon the present scarce supply of psychiatrists. It is essential that individual psychiatrists learn to support and consult with people who really reach low-income families, and are therefore better able to assist them.

It is lamentable that neither Washington nor Ottawa have real information relating to overall mental health needs. In both countries, the most serious bottleneck to progress in mental health revolves around the lack of adequate facilities and the fact that most departments of psychiatry are removed from the general hospital. The lack of psychiatric facilities and personnel is typified in the New York City area, where there was found to be a one-year waiting list for children needing pediatric psychiatric service.

Psychiatric hospitals should be called Community Health Centres. Mental illness or breakdown should be faced up to for what it is. A greater segment of the population must be involved, so that problems are recognized early and prevention is underlined.

Dr. Leonard J. Duhl, Chief, Office of Planning, National Institute of Mental Health, United States Public Health Service, feels that, together with other professions, psychiatry will have to keep judging the community from the standpoint of its own knowledge and findings. Only by this means, can it help to formulate the instruments which will promote mental health and wholeness.

Death On Our Roads

There is one last disease I should mention: The epidemic of automobile and highway deaths and injuries.

On September 13, 1899, H. H. Bliss, a New York City real estate agent, was returning home from a successful business meeting late in the afternoon. Stepping down from a trolly bus at the corner of Central Park West and 74th Street, Bliss was struck and killed by an automobile. He became the first of millions to lose his life by the automobile. Now in just a single year, 59,000 North Americans die on the highways. In Canada, we kill well over 5,000 every year, with another annual toll of 210,000 permanently disabled. Every second car rolling off the assembly line will be involved in a death or injury, producing accident.

Automobile and highway deaths and injuries constitute a worldwide public health problem, an epidemic involving the vehicle, the driver, the road and the surroundings. In North America, this is the biggest killer of our young people under thirty-five; the third largest killer of all our people after heart disease and cancer. Since Mr. Bliss was killed before the turn of the century, more North Americans have died on our roads than all the victims of all our wars in all our history. The private and public sectors, co-operating with all levels of government, must mobilize the conscience of our people and the technology of our times to end the senseless slaughter of the mechanized age.

Ottawa and Washington must set up National Accident Prevention Research Centres, and also draw up "meaningful" rules to recall dangerous cars from the roads, as well as setting "meaningful" safety performance standards for vehicles at the manufacturing level. All levels of government must design and build better and safer roads. Our States, provinces and municipalities, must police and educate better and safer drivers, while ordering a "meaningful" and regular inspection for vehicles already on the road, as well as the safety certification of second-hand vehicles before re-sale.

In Canada and the United States, accidents in general, and highway and motor vehicle accidents in particular, are viewed largely as being inevitable. Their prevention is given a low national priority on both sides of the border. This lack of public concern, imagination and initiative can sometimes be excused on the grounds of ignorance. Official foot-dragging on the part of government officials, both elected and appointed, who know what is needed, is another story. It is another part of the cynical story of our North American institutions, institutions which fail to respond to decent and legitimate demands, institutions which continue to alienate more and more thinking North Americans.

If a conclusion to this chapter is valid, it is that a great deal of effort needs to be expended on curing the diseases of affluence, such as unsafe motor vehicles, dirty water, and dirty air. Preventive medicine must mean more than regular checkups or safety on the job. It must constitute a dedicated and sustained assault by all members of our society against these diseases of affluence which, unchecked, threaten to make all other disease obsolete.

15
Quackery, Occult Healing and Near-Medicine

If a crisis occurs in your treatment, insist vehemently, there is no disease, there can be no pain.
MARY BAKER EDDY, FOUNDER OF THE CHURCH OF CHRIST SCIENTIST

In the eighteenth century, Dr. Elisha Perkins with his "metallic tractors" was, perhaps, the first quack to put a significant product on the North American market. His metal rods supposedly pulled diseases from the body, and he gained recognition and support from George Washington, Chief Justice Marshall of the Supreme Court and many other of the Capitol's first leaders. Since that time, panacea has followed panacea and the nostrum peddlers have grown more cunning. As technology advanced, electricity and radio were employed to defraud an unsuspecting public. Dr. Ruth B. Drown's radio therapy instrument came on the market in the early nineteen thirties, and according to Drown could treat people by remote control. Dr. Drown had never attended a medical school and her experience in radio had developed through building a crystal set.

In 1966, the annual quackery take in the United States and Canada was estimated at more than two billion dollars. Quackery and self-dosage still thrive in North America because of the failure of our system to deliver legitimate health and medical care services and the resulting unfulfilled promise to many members of our society. Into the vacuum moves the quack with cruel and costly results.

There are great difficulties in regulating quackery. The first is that most people simply refuse to admit they have been taken. In any event, the dividing line between quackery and real medicine was always unclear because most practices of medicine which were acceptable at one time are now considered to be quackery.

Quackery thrives because of ignorance. A series of suggestions and counter-suggestions presented by the quack often create an illness where none existed before. Personality structure has much to do with susceptibility to the practice and many who opt for quackery do so in a beligerently anti-intellectual manner. Terrible poverty in many North American cities has produced strong anti-intellectual characteristics and the quack with his good "common sense" seems far superior to the expert professionals. Yet, intellectuals, too, get trapped occasionally. University towns all over North America are hot-beds of quackery. Nonetheless, it is the poor in education and means who take the biggest soaking.

Still, further forces are at work. If you have arthritis you may eventually try anything to relieve the painful condition. Also, a physicians's therapy may often be unpleasant as is sometimes the case with insulin treatments. Through the centuries, the quack has played on the deep-rooted suspicion of regular doctors as some people go through life carrying the mystical and magical concepts of their youth. It must also be said that several individuals who were treated as quacks in their lifetimes turned out to be proponents of valid theories. These exceptions afford small comfort when compared to the pitiful toll heaped upon North American society by dollar-orientated charlatans who prey on suffering, frustration and hopelessness.

The main aim of quackery was and is "the fast buck" and as long as the causes of disease are a mystery even to doctors, the critique of quackery cannot be completely persuasive.

J. F. Kelly and "Mental Healing"

There are significant cases which highlight the story of quackery in North America. In 1897, United States postal authorities became suspicious of the activities of a mental healing practitioner, J. H. Kelly. Kelly had settled in Nevada, Missouri, where he soon began practicing and teaching. He incorporated a venture under the name "American School of Magnetic Healing." Besides face-to-face treatment, he emphasized treatments at a distance. The human mind, so he claimed, was mainly responsible for sickness. The patient therefore had to clear his mind of all disturbing thoughts at the moment the transmittor in Nevada despatched a cure. By 1900, three thousand letters a day were arriving in Nevada for the Magnetic School. The school's daily take ran from one thousand to sixteen hundred dollars. The post office stopped the mail as fraudulent, but the courts intervened on Kelly's behalf. Justice Peckham of the Supreme Court ruled in favour of Kelly, and incredibly extended his argument to the whole field of therapy, creating a massive roadblock to controlling quackery. Said Peckham, "The influence of the mind upon the physical condition of the body is very powerful and a hopeful mental state goes far, in many cases, not only to alleviate but even to aid very largely in the case of an illness from which the body may suffer." However true this may have been, certainly such a general doctrine should not have provided an escape hatch for Kelly and subsequent practitioners of quackery.

Another discouraging fact began to be evident to those within the Post Office Department charged with combatting public fraud. Some quacks were virtually impossible to curb. Defeated in one venture, they started another with a new name, a new address, and often with a new and more sophisticated and devious approach.

Albert Abrams and "Spondyclotherapy"

To many, Albert Abrams, with his notions of "electronic reactions" is the dean of twentieth century charlatans. In 1890, Abrams became a professor of pathology at the Cooper Medical College in San Francisco. His theory of healing was called "Spondyclotherapy." According to Abrams, he could diagnose disease and cure it too by a steady and rapid percussion or hammering of the spine. He also "percussed" the abdomen, and soon his new approach and theory became gadget-orientated, implementing electricity and radio for diagnosis. His assortment of devices supposedly detected syphillis, T.B., and cancer and the "exact" location of the disease. Then came his Oscilloclast, capable of producing vibrations in consonance with the vibratory rates of all known diseases. Abrams died from pneumonia at the age of 60 while under heavy attack from a special committee set up by the *Scientific American*. He left an estate valued at $2,000,000.

The end of the Second World War and the huge surplus of electrical equipment on the market saw a proportionate increase in device quackery. It meant a deluge of Oscillators, Electropads, Radioclasts, Neurolinometors, Micro Dynameters and other devices. In 1964, Washington's Food and Drug Act Commissioner, George Larrick stated, "So many fake gadgets are still in the hands of practitioners that if we set all of our inspectors at work on nothing else it would take several years to find and take successful action against all these devices."

Before the sixties, many anti-quackery journalistic crusades had commenced and in October, 1961, a National Congress on Medical Quackery in the United States was held. Seven hundred men and women came from State medical societies and licensing boards. The

131

question of "rigged research" came in for much criticism. "Rigged research" was described as a study set up and written to support a claim, rather than to seek scientific proof. Speaker after speaker at the conference heaped criticisms on newspapers and magazines for flamboyant stories about unfounded medical advances which were just specious promotions. The conference noted that quackery channels more than 2 per cent of the United States national budget into the hands of criminals. Cancer quackery is the leader, and quackery in general is a criminal activity as harmful as any in society but against which Washington and Ottawa does the least. North American regulation is not only meaningless but virtually non-existent.

As we said, the dividing line between quackery and medicine is often blurred but let's look now at some quasi-medical areas where there is cause for grave doubts.

Occult Healers

Many of these individuals frame their doctrines in the language of the natural sciences. According to them spirits flow "like an electric current from positive to negative poles." To many, nineteenth-century occult healing virtually meant "mind cure." You merely concentrated on the perfect reality of health, prosperity, success and happiness. Occult healing has tended to move into an area where medicine is notoriously ill-equipped to cope: that of emotional disorders and psychological distress. Added to this is the fact that thousands crave personal contact with healers, not impersonal treatment. Increasing sophistication and intellectualization of the older and more orthodox churches has led to a great lack of personal warmth and contact in people's lives.

Hypnosis and Hypnotherapy

Any discussion of occult healing soon involves the whole field of hypnosis and hypnotherapy. Mesmer set up the first secular practice in Paris in 1778, based on his theories of "animal magnetism." Towards the end of the nineteenth century a French neurologist, Jean-Martin Charcot, demonstrated the therapeutic use of hypnosis, and in 1882, the French Academy of Medicine officially recognized the legitimate medical use of hypnosis. Another seventy-five years passed before the British, American and Canadian medical associations followed suit.

It must be said that hypnosis has a constructive place in modern medicine, especially in treatment of habit-type sicknesses with underlying psychological disorders such as alcoholism, smoking and obesity. Painless childbirth is another example of its successful application.

Yet hypnosis, as such, is not a therapy. Patients are treated "under" hypnosis not "with" it. In 1963, less than 4 per cent of North American physicians used hypnosis, and no Canadian medical school, for example, offers training in the subject.

Nevertheless, the dangers of hypnosis should not be overlooked. The first danger or risk is that it is impossible to accurately predict what specific phenomena will occur when any given subject is hypnotized. An untrained and incompetent hypnotist may find himself called upon to handle problems for which he is not equipped. Secondly, there are certain spontaneous phenomena which appear in some subjects without their being suggested and for no apparent reason. Amnesia, catelepsy, and even hallucinations may occur. Another danger may occur when hypnotherapy is used to treat only the symptoms of what is in fact a serious organic disorder. Also, the incompetent use of hypnosis may have other effects resulting from failure to completely remove any unwanted suggestions accidentally induced during hypnosis. For example, a poor hypnotist may panic and cannot wake a patient up, and, again, the attempt to induce hypnosis may itself precipitate a severe psychological reaction such as hysteria, convulsions and uncontrollable fits of laughter or crying.

According to the Report of the Committee on the Healing Arts, regulation of hypnotherapists is far from adequate. In the yellow pages of a Toronto telephone book under the listing "Family and Marriage Counsellors and Hypnotists" one practitioner's degrees are listed, all gained at the Philathea College of London, Ontario, between 1961 and 1966. The college is a private corporation which the Ontario Department of University Affairs describes as unrecommended and which the Association of Universities and Colleges of Canada lists as "unaccredited."

Lack of suitable training facilities in hypnotherapy for physicians remains one of the major bottle-necks and the American Medical Association has produced a detailed course programme. The A.M.A. suggests a "hypnosis technician" could operate only under a professionally qualified therapist.

In Ontario, the *Hypnosis Act* forbids the practice of hypnosis by any person, except by a physician, a dentist, or psychologist under the direction of a physician or such persons as may be permitted under the regulations. The regulations, on the other hand, permit lay practitioners to remain in practice if they have earned at least $2,500 in five years of practice before 1961. California courts have already issued an interpretation including hypnotherapy as part of the practice of medicine.

Electropsychometry and its practice is a specialized application of hypnosis. It was the invention of the recently deceased Volney G. Mathison of California, a renowned hypnotist who claimed some skills in electronics which he applied to the E-Meter. He called it the X-Ray of the human psyche. He would use it, he said, to accurately pin-point traumatic areas of the patient's psyche. He claimed his method was "a new way to a capable, successful, serene self." For instance a practitioner of electropsychometry in Toronto is a regularly qualified naturopath and physiotherapist who says he holds a P.L.D. in metaphysics from the Universal College of Truth in Chicago obtained by correspondence. The college, which was never accredited, is now defunct. There is absolutely no regulation of his practice, even though the E-Meter can in no way be considered as the X-Ray of the human psyche.

Concept Therapy is yet another secular system of healings which bears investigation. It incorporates self-hypnosis with a variety of scientific doctrines and invention of a chiropractor, Dr. Thomas Fleet of San Antonio, Texas. He began teaching the concept in 1931. Concept therapy argues only 20 per cent of all human ailments need to be treated by surgery, drugs and other means; the remaining 80 per cent are psychosomatic. Graduates of Concept Therapy classes are called "Beamers." They are "on the beam" of the consciousness which runs through all reality. All club officers are named after members of an air crew. Thus, there is no president but a captain, a navigator, gunner, and so on. A promotional ad for the concept ran this way, "What is it worth for you to learn how to better defend against thoughts which may cause cancer, ulcers, severe tooth ailments, appendicitis and the like?"

Faith Healing

Whether "faith healing" can be termed occult is an open question, yet it is one that demands examination here. The First Church of Christ Scientist is a century-old Protestant denomination of American origin founded by Mrs. Mary Baker Eddy. The healing of all forms of illness and distress of its members is the major goal and activity of the church. Its healing is founded on the metaphysical doctrine that all material substance, including the human body, is completely unreal. The Christian Science Church claims that physicians actually promote human suffering by diagnosing disease.

The Church has always sought to avoid regulation of its healing aspects through constitutional guarantees of the freedom of religion. However, in Ontario, the Church appealed recently to the Workmen's Compensation Board for a recognition of its practitioners which would be equivalent to that granted the medical profession. Although presented as part of their religious beliefs, healing has always been the central activity of Christian Science. Their doctrine supports the idea that "to material sense, the severance of the jugular vein takes away life, but to spiritual sense, and in Science life, things go on unchanged and being is eternal. Temporal life is a false sense of existence." The psychological doctrine of Christian Science argues that the human body is unreal. At one point the Church felt that even adherence to the laws of hygiene was useless. Originally, Mrs. Eddy taught "metaphysical obstetrics," eliminating medical attention at birth, but this was dropped in 1901 after the death of a mother and daughter.

The Christian Science practitioner does offer services to the general public, not just members of the Church, so we must ask how he is trained, recruited, accredited and disciplined. Full-time practitioners charge fees, but no practitioner gets a patient's history or keeps records. Their treatment is still largely effected by Mrs. Eddy's dictum, "If a crisis occurs in your treatment, insist, vehemently, there is no disease, there can be no pain."

Does it work? Well, consider a couple of the cases described in the *Committee of the Healing Arts* report. For example, there was the Christian Science schoolteacher who made sworn affidavits for several consecutive years that she was free from infectious disease, although being treated by a practitioner for "living congestion." When she finally entered a hospital she died in one day from tuberculosis. Or consider the worker in an ordnance plant who had an accident while moving a vat of concentrated acid. Some of it splashed in his right eye. Later he declared, "My first impulse was to get to a water faucet and wash my eye, but I knew I could not afford to admit even by this simple act that an accident or evil can befall God's man."

Christian Science is recognized by some social security and medicare legislation of the United States and both the u.s. and Canadian federal governments . accept receipts of practitioners' fees for income tax deductions. Only eighteen states and no Canadian provinces have recognized Christian Science under Workmen's Compensation legislation. As far as regulation is concerned, there is no restriction on healing by prayer and spiritual means, but most areas in North America require adherence to public health laws. Thus, members of the Church accepted smallpox immunization.

Then, of course, there is Oral Roberts, a Pentecostal, perhaps the best known faith healer in North America. His crusades visit many cities and those seeking his intercession with God are urged to "expect a miracle." He wants to cast out demons. His familiar cry of "In the name of Jesus Christ, be healed! Be healed! Be healed!" is still heard regularly over radio and television across North America.

In 1925, A. C. Gabelein studied three hundred and fifty persons who received treatment from a faith healer in Vancouver. He found 301 patients had no change, 39 died within six months, 5 became mentally ill and 5 were cured. Physicians said the cures had a normal medical explanation.

Faith healing practices on the part of the Toronto Anglican "Demon Cult" at Saint Mathias Anglican Church in downtown Toronto in 1967 came in for much publicity. A group at the church practiced the exorcism of demons. In September 1967, an inquest was held into the death of one of its members. The inquest found that the Anglican priest and his wife had been negligent in the death of an eighteen-year-old girl, a member of the occult group and a resident in the church rectory as the legal ward of the priest. She died in June, 1967, from a brain abcess and meningitis. At one time she was continually screaming and the priest believed she was possessed of the devil. At the inquest the priest admitted that his religious beliefs had clouded his judgement, and that he had believed his ward's trouble to be only emotional. He spanked her ritually. When the girl's body was removed to the coroner's morgue, three members of the group went to the morgue and prayed over her body. Lazarus, they noted, had been called from the dead two thousand years before.

Dianetics and Scientology

Dianetics and Scientology constitute the next stage for investigation in occult practices. To some, Dianetics is "the modern science of mental health" and was spearheaded by L. Ron Hubbard. He is an Ameri-

136

can science fiction writer who claimed he was a graduate engineer. He is not. Hubbard is a doctor of philosophy from an unaccredited California university. He also is a doctor of Scientology, a degree he awarded himself when he founded Scientology. Scientology claims to be a religion "a spiritual guide designed to bring about total freedom to all spiritual beings." Dianetics and Scientology are inseparable according to Hubbard. "Eye glasses, nervous twitches, tension, all of these things stem from an unwillingness to confront. When that unwillingness is repaired, these disabilities tend to disappear." Hubbard claimed his treatment "alleviates burns received from Atomic Bombs and is a method of preventing mental derangement." Scientology is extremely antagonistic to the medical profession particularly towards psychiatrists. Like Mrs. Eddy, Hubbard is quite concerned to protect his own personal interest in the commercial propagation of his teachings. For example, all information materials received by a student remain the property of Hubbard.

Hubbard published his first book, *Dianetics, The Modern Science of Mental Health* in 1950. In February, 1952, his Dianetic Research Foundation went bankrupt after New Jersey authorities charged its auditors with illegally practicing medicine. He then moved to Kansas but the movement dissolved. Next Hubbard and friends hurriedly got together the "electropsychrometer" or "E-Meter." One of its claims was a cure for cancer. Setting up his headquarters in Phoenix, Arizona, Hubbard got in behind the religious front establishing "The Church of Scientology of California and of Washington." In 1962 the Food and Drug administration seized one hundred E-Meters from the Washington Scientology offices. Yet, Scientology continues to legally operate under Hubbard on five continents, sometimes with pitiful results.

There is no instance of favourable recognition in the Western World for Scientology, yet in North America there is absolutely no regulation. Objective experimental verification of Hubbard's physiological and psychological doctrines is lacking, and Scientology only took on a religious form after it suffered a severe set-back as a "science of mental health."

Spiritualist Healing is yet another occult practice which poses many basic problems. The operative agency involved in Spiritualist Healing is a spirit or bands of spirits of former living persons, in particular the spirits of great physicians of the past. Healing as a part of spiritualist practice did not become prevalent until the twentieth century. Today, at a typical Christian Spiritualist Healing Club in

North America, the patient goes to the healing chair. The healer dips his hands in water in a nearby basin, rubs them together vigorously and grasps the patient firmly by the shoulders near the neck, standing behind the chair. A formula is repeated, for example, "I of myself can do nothing, but through God all things are possible." After several minutes the healer moves his hands to the head of the patient and finally grasps the hands firmly. He bows his head, prays and dismisses the patient. The positive power of the spirit should never be minimized, but claims for spiritual healing have included cures for spinal problems and arthritis. The dangers of current widespread non-regulation are obvious.

The Patent Medicine Racket

It is impossible to write about quackery without mentioning patent medicines. After all, the patent medicine man is part of our folklore and was a familiar sight in towns and villages a hundred years ago. Miracles were his stock in trade – although he often left town in a hurry. Family fortunes were built on patent medicines and they continue to be built today.

Perhaps the king of the modern medicine men was Dudley J. Leblanc, a state senator from Louisiana who promoted Hadacol, an elixir of 12 per cent alcohol, plus some of the **B** complex vitamins, iron, calcium, phosphorous, dilute hydrochloric acid, and honey. Leblanc mixed the first batches in big barrels behind his Abberville, Louisiana, barn and nearby farmers' daughters stirred it with boat oars.

In 1950, Hadacol grossed at least twenty million dollars within its sales area of twenty-two states. Toward the close of the year, Leblanc's advertising bill was a fat one million dollars per month, taking in about seven hundred daily papers, four thousand seven hundred weeklies and five hundred and twenty-eight radio stations. According to Leblanc, Hadacol would "restore youthful feeling and appearance" and it would ensure "good health." Claims for Hadacol knew no bounds. Leblanc recreated the old-fashioned medicine show, and in the summer of 1950 a caravan of one hundred and thirty vehicles toured the South. Dixieland bands played "Hadacol Boogie" and "Who Put The Pep In Grandma?" What was Hadacol good for? This question was put to Leblanc by Groucho Marx on television, "Hadacol" replied Leblanc smilingly, "was good for five and a half million for me last year."

138

Soon Leblanc sold his interests in Hadacol, but the whole enterprise had become overextended and the new owners went into bankruptcy, while federal authorities finally caught up with Leblanc. The Hadacol bubble had burst.

Sensitivity Groups and "Near Medicine"

Today in some regions, we are moving out of the strict area of occult healing into what could be termed at times, an equally dangerous practice of near-medicine. In various North American cities "mind-blowing sensitivity weekends" are the "in" thing. These weekends involve group therapy, usually conducted by untrained people, and often include emotionally disturbed as well as normal individuals. Without regulation, it is impossible to ascertain what damage or good is ultimately done both to the disturbed and non-disturbed. Five hundred "human potential" groups involving five thousand people have sprung up in Toronto. Some sources say as many as twenty thousand Torontonians are considering joining one. The group "leaders," "trainees," or "facilitators" all make the general claim to attempt to expand human awareness without the use of drugs. Regulation, for many reasons, seems a must, as many of the groups have taken on a commercial nature. One Canadian company is a case in point. There are approximately four hundred and fifty members paying seventy-five to eighty-five dollars per month into it. The company owns many houses and an apartment building. It also owns a nearby farm, valued at more than half a million dollars.

The whole question of these groups involves the untrained, unlicensed individual taking the place, too often, of the trained psychologist, psychiatrist, hypnotist, and of general psychological therapy to persons in need of professional help.

The sensitivity session often involves members of a group examining one fellow member to discover all his faults and point out what they do not like about him. The session usually emphasizes the breaking down of normal social relationships in order to achieve what is termed "maximum expression and inter-action between group members." There are a number of serious ramifications for the innocent persons participating in group therapy in search of help for emotional, social and mental disturbances. The dilemma is further complicated when it is not only the lay therapist who is involved, but several other group members often suffering from varying degrees of mental

139

problems. More precisely, such therapy keeps people from seeking recognized qualified help because they have found a crutch.

Although there is general disapproval in the medical profession of many of these groups, no active steps have been taken to curtail their activities. The same is true of the Better Business Bureau and, at present in Canada, there are no municipal, provincial or federal laws pertaining to this field. It is, of course, difficult and probably wrong to control people who are simply voluntarily getting together to solve their own personal problems. It is a matter of individual freedom. However, consumer protection should be achieved whenever financial exchange is involved. Needed are standards permitting licensing and regulatory controls to be exercised to protect the individual from the potential injustices of the group structure. Secondly, in such cases where, in fact, medical practices are taking place, strict regulatory controls should be obligatory and, thirdly, where fraudulent and corrupt business practices are taking place, similarly strict legal sanctions are a must. In addition officials both in government and in the social and medical fields should attempt to educate the public as to the serious dangers of such groups.

Yet yesterday's legitimate medicine is often today's quackery, and yesterday's quackery invariably attains a high degree of respectability and legitimacy with the passage of time. Modern medicine is taking another look at magnetism for example. This mainstay of quackery for generations has long been ignored by doctors. Nevertheless, early in 1970 a group of scientists from seven countries met at the Weizmann Institute of Science in Rehovat, Israel, to reconsider magnetism as a medical aid. They reviewed an array of magnetic devices that were possibly useful for treating inaccessible aneurysms, getting drugs to certain parts of the brain, measuring blood flow to tiny vessels, picking up a magnetic whisper from a silent heart valve and by-passing blind spots of the electrocardiogram. They saw how magnetic devices could move an intestine out of the way during radiation of a neighbouring organ. While these considerations are obviously valid, it is no argument for allowing the devious and commercially-orientated quack to continue to offer fake and dangerous "cures" to an uninformed and unprotected public. Even the broadest interpretation of commercial laissez-faire does not allow for such activity.

Freedom of religion makes it difficult to regulate many areas of occult healing and, again, it should be emphasized that the power of faith and the spirit should never be minimized even with regard to physical and mental well being. But, those who hide behind religious

140

facades in order to foster fake healing practices for commercial ends should be recognized for what they are, ferreted out, policed and regulated.

Education and regulation are key words to be remembered in any attempt to control quackery, occult healing and near-medicine. Education and regulations are listed in that order for it is questionable how much regulation can protect an uninformed public.

Quackery flourishes when high expectations remain unfulfilled, when cures long since available are not being delivered on a broad and equitable basis to all the people. The implications are obvious. Until our collapsing system of legitimate health and medical services is updated and humanized, unregulated North American quackery will take an ever-increasing toll.

16
Conclusion

Health and wellbeing are available here and now, and are the people's right and not by grace, chance, nor fortune.
DR. JOHN MALONEY

Hippocrates, the Father of Medicine, wrote a code of medical ethics which included some eighty-seven treatises. An oath of allegiance to ethical professional standards, they were imposed on his disciples, and that same oath, in one form or another, must still be taken by men about to enter medical practice.

However Hippocrates died in 377 B.C., and today his fine words and lofty sentiments are not of much assistance to a modern doctor, who is attempting to cope realistically with the demands of contemporary society. For example, when Dr. Christian Barnard, the South African surgeon, began transplanting hearts from those who had just died to those whose hearts would soon fail them, he unwittingly posed a new moral question for the medical professions of the world: At what point *is* someone medically dead? Other questions, such as sterilization and abortion, have brought the medical world face to face with the need to rewrite their code of ethics, as did the Canadian Medical Association in 1970.

Whether our images come to us from books or movies portraying times past, the white-aproned pharmacist measuring out his chemicals from jars, the medical doctor making a house call late at night, or even the much celebrated and heroic efforts of nurses such as Florence Nightingale, all contrast sharply with our contemporary impressions of the big city hospital with its vast array of expensive scientific equipment and highly trained staff.

The contrast is clear when one goes back to the beginning of medicine's history in North America. When Louis Hébert arrived at Quebec village in 1617, where he was to be the doctor for the ensuing decade, he planted what were reputed to be the first crops along the shores of the St. Lawrence. He had great success as a farmer as well as a doctor and in the course of practising his limited and perfunctory medicine, he was able to help feed many people who otherwise would have gone hungry. Today we seem to expect virtually everything from doctors – with the possible exception of a sack of potatoes to help us through a long winter. This phenomenon can be seen throughout North America. Only recently have the leaders of organized medicine reluctantly recognized the fact that North Americans regard decent health and medical care as one of their rights, not a privilege, or a commodity to be sold by medical men on the open market.

In November of 1969, Dr. John Maloney, Chairman of a Canadian government task force enquiring into methods of delivering medical care, had made much the same point from the doctors side of the fence. Maloney spoke of an "increasing conviction of the people that health and wellbeing are available here and now and are theirs by right and not by grace, chance, nor fortune."

A variety of factors have caused this expanded demand in the past decade: increasing affluence, new infusions of purchasing power, private and public insurance schemes, more education, more awareness of health, rapid growth in the youngest and oldest segments of the population, continuing urbanization, and, as I said in an earlier chapter, an increasingly sensitive social consciousness. Just as the theological philosophy of medieval man was replaced by the rationalistic philosophy of the eighteenth and nineteenth centuries, so was this in turn replaced by the man-centered or humanistic philosophy of today. Political leaders, for example, when discussing the medical situation, frequently express the conviction that the health resources of our country, its personnel facilities and money, should be mainly oriented to those who are poor, remote or disadvantaged; to those who in the past have not benefited as much as society's privileged few.

Accompanying this new social sensitivity is an increasing readiness to turn to science for the answers to more and more of our human problems. Alcoholism and other addictions, personality disorders, criminal tendencies and many other problems that in the past have not been thought of as medical ones will increasingly be dumped into medicine's lap for a solution. These pressures will create a demand for new and better procedures and, as an illustration, Dr. Maloney cites three areas of medicine where a great deal more will be expected.

First is the one-organ death. An otherwise vigorous man with a bad heart, or failing kidneys, or cirrhotic liver, will look to a transplant to put him back on the fully active list. The number of older people in our country is increasing, due to greater longevity and the general aging of our population, and as a consequence there are more degenerative diseases. Added to this is the fact that much of the basic work on organ replacement has been done and artificial organs are being developed, and one can quickly see what extensive and expensive

143

medical services will be demanded by this large and influential group of citizens, with their demand for artificial hearts, kidneys, livers, arteries, hip-joints, and so on.

Secondly, there will be increased expectations in constructive and cosmetic surgery. What is being done now with big ears and crooked noses is only a beginning and soon medicine will be called upon for such tasks as slicing off double chins, cutting off pot bellies and transplanting hair.

Thirdly, there will be increasing pressure for better results in the treatment of cancer. It is probable, for several reasons, that this will show itself first in the case of cancer of the breast, a tragically common disease. It often hits when the family is young and vulnerable, and the survival rate under present treatments has not increased appreciably for 30 or 40 years. Recent research indicates that the traditional treatment, disfiguring amputation, is neither satisfactory nor always necessary.

Other developments, such as concern about over-population combined with the desire to bring healthier children into the world, as well as far greater efforts in the area of preventative medicine and public health, will also place new demands on medicine. More extensive medical services are now being required in both genetic counselling and birth control programmes for sterilization and abortion.

Many of these subjects emerged from under the table at the hundred-and-third Annual Meeting of the Canadian Medical Association in Winnipeg in the spring of 1970. A new code of ethics was approved, replacing some of those guidelines set down by Hippocrates. Significantly, the new code makes no mention at all of abortion. It was felt that abortion should be regarded in the same way as any other surgical procedure – in the light of whether it was for the well-being of the patient. Another major change, organ transplantation, was also recognized for the first time in the new code. These advances, and the free and open discussion of such questions as sterilization, surprised some observers as being not only unprecedented but remarkably progressive for the Canadian Medical Association. Yet, while hopefully a sign of the times, the change in attitude was, typically, long overdue. The new president of the c.m.a., Dr. D. L. Kippen, is certainly cognizant of the new pressures on the medical profession. His expressed opinions reflect the inevitable shift in attitudes that have taken place beneath the surface. Says Kippen, "Organized medicine has had to take into consideration legal, social and at times political matters before it can make a statement on policy. What we are seeing now is a more liberal attitude in society in general, and the doctors are moving with the times. These changed attitudes have not been effected overnight."

Nor have they come about in a vacuum. As the demand for medical services started racing ahead at an ever-increasing velocity, and as the ability of medicine to produce miraculous new results increased, the state could remain a spectator for only so long. Almost inevitably the political process was called upon to intervene, to ensure that distribution of the medical facilities available was equitable and fair for all of society. As Canada and the United States of America embraced more and more aspects of the Welfare State, either consciously or unconsciously, a new concept became part of our conventional, everyday attitudes. Slowly we came to accept the idea that government should take the responsibility of providing a minimum level of health and medical care and medical assistance, by paying doctor and hospital bills.

Of course the United Kingdom had already established the necessary precedent. The National Health Service has been in existence there since 1949, and today it is almost impossible to find an opponent of "socialized medicine" left on the island. Of course, there are still critics of the Health Service: doctors who are discouraged and bitter; patients who complain loudly and frequently; individuals who would not dream of accepting free state medical treatment, and physicians who will have nothing to do with state-paid medical practice. But no one *really* wants to turn back the clock two decades and return to the old medical systems. Indeed, long before the advent of the National Health Service, government legislation had, in a piece-meal way, struggled over a period of years to implement a more modern and progressive approach to the country's medical needs.

In Canada, the movement toward the same end was slower but just as inevitable. Our first recognition of the need for government to take an active role in guaranteeing adequate medical and health services came in 1958, with the Hospital Insurance programme. A further necessary step came eleven years later, in 1969, when the Medical Insurance programme was implemented.

The government-operated Hospital Insurance programme is far-reaching. All provinces now provide hospital out-patient services on an emergency basis, as well as in-patient services at the standard, or public ward level.

The second big change, Medical Insurance, resulted in a compulsory, comprehensive state-operated medical insurance programme covering doctor's charges. Medicare in North America had already been pioneered by the c.c.f. government in Saskatchewan in 1962, which had afterwards resulted in a doctor's "strike," but the handwriting was on the wall. By 1969 it became obvious that the public wanted government-paid medical care and that doctors must learn to accept it as an inescapable fact of life.

American governments – both state and federal – have continued to assume a larger and larger role in providing and paying for the health and care of its citizens. As far back as the days of the "New Deal," there was a rapid acceleration of this process, although at other times opposition, from such groups as the American Medical Association which opposes "the strangling of medicine in government and red tape," were so well organized and effective that the two rival schools of thought achieved a complete deadlock. Nevertheless the trend has continued, and now the United States has both Medicare and Medicaid. Expenditures in these and related programmes soar into the billions annually.

And, as I said earlier, there's the rub. We can all agree that progress is inevitable, and, indeed desirable. But progress, by definition, means an increasing complexity in the structure of society, and an apparently endless acceleration of costs and services.

This acceleration is not occurring in a vacuum. It is part of an entire matrix of problems facing North American society today. The only solution lies in a co-ordinated effort which must take place at all levels of society.

By definition, this seems like an almost impossible aim. What possible means can be found to get government, the public, industry and doctors to work together? Yet those means must be found if we are to clean up the present mess.

As a first step we must stop looking at the "bits," the hospital, doctors, nurses, the delivery system, the financing mechanism, and so on – as independent factors. They must be co-ordinated to provide adequate care for all persons who need it. The major need is for national health systems to establish policies for co-ordinating the health and medical requirements of North Americans. Four major areas require greater efficiency: the individual facility, the community, the state, as well as provincial and national levels.

This means more organization, planning and control at all these levels. Such elements have long since been introduced into the indus-

146

trial system, and must be quickly introduced into North American medical and health care services.

The kind of massive reorganization necessary only becomes possible if we establish "systems" controls.

The systems approach has been remarkably successful in weapons development and space programs. Why can it not be applied to the problems of medical and health care services? The systems approach looks for specific solutions to specific problems, and at the same time demands justification for the existence of any programme within a set of programmes, and for each element within each programme. A "systems" approach requires immediate action within many specific areas. What are some of these areas in the field of medicine?

The Role of the Government

Medical and health care services constitute just one of the many challenges which are *not* being met by federalism as now practiced in both Canada and the United States. Like the challenge of the environment, transportation and living space in our cities, education and the rest, medical and health care services test the very viability of North American federalism. If North American Medicare and Medicaid schemes continue merely to be a "finance mechanism," the complete breakdown of services will come about sooner than we care to think. If doctor's incomes continue to soar, government authorities will have to put them on salaries. If doctors and medical manpower won't go into underserviced areas, surely a decent and humane state has an obligation to make sure medical personnel is equitably deployed. Public costs means that public resources should be used to influence the operation of "systems" that are essential for the health needs of all the people. Costs will continue to skyrocket if governments, working with the public and medical profession, do not assume their responsibilities in determining that the plant, personnel and services are made "ready." If they are not, what was the money voted for in the first place?

Governments' relationship with business must also alter. Modern free enterprise has conferred enormous benefits upon North Americans, and will continue to do so, but when only a very few corporate giants ruin things for the vast majority of us, government must step in, draw up and enforce the ground rules.

147

The Role of the Small Community

Ottawa and Washington must give strong central direction and co-ordination to their programs, but the delivery of modern medical and health care services means a high degree of decentralization, which in turn means responsiveness to local and community needs. Washington and Ottawa don't have all the answers. More often, local people and local communities know what is best for themselves and how best to govern their affairs. At the same time, the central authority must assure local action is carried out in co-operation with other regions.

To date, Washington and Ottawa have not taken account of the principle of "local self agency." Forcing the states and provinces to participate in Medicare schemes, both federal authorities are doing next to nothing to permit the states, provinces, and, in turn, local governments to have realistic taxing powers in order to play their part in any progressive Medicaid or Medicare programme. By refusing to help make ready the plant, resources and personnel for these programmes, Washington and Ottawa must share much of the blame for the current nightmare.

If we are serious about a better and more equitable distribution of services, especially in the doctorless villages of rural and inner core urban areas, immediate action is necessary. More regional clinics will have to be built together with smaller clinics in local communities. Family health workers will have to be trained in order to work with-doctors and local people. For all paramedical workers a uniform standard of subsidization for their training should be implemented together with a proper quality control supervising system. We need a continuous flow of well-motivated, qualified workers. This means the successful application of incentives and career planning. Medical schools and hospitals with community and regional responsibilities should have the task of creating a sytematic scheme for recruiting, training and deploying the paramedical worker.

Hospitals

Sound management and business techniques must be applied to hospitals. These include staff organization and effective communications, "meaningful" financial reporting, regional planning, effective utilization of manpower, and computer technology. Objective criteria must be set up for admissions, investigations and treatment, length of stay and discharge. Doctors must realize the financial considerations of their activities.

No longer can we allow our hospitals to be doctors' workshops. Incentives to improve care, reduce costs and improve efficiencies must be introduced within the hospital sector. Administrators, not doctors, must run our hospitals. Trustees and governors should be responsible for over-all policy, and doctors must concentrate upon the practice of medicine.

In the future, regional hospital planning must receive more emphasis as hospitals assume more responsibilities toward the particular communities in which they are to be found. A greater number of hospitals will have to share high-cost facilities. Hospital admissions will be reduced only if we give proper priority to expenditures for preventative medicine, health care clinics, general ambulatory care centres, home care programmes, regional and community clinics, nursing and convalescent homes and other facilities that could treat and care for patients who now find themselves admitted to general community hospitals.

In the area of discipline and control relating to hospitals, Ottawa and Washington must assume responsibility for the adequate staffing and financing of accreditation programmes. Peer review and medical auditing must be made meaningful, while medical record procedures are updated with the help of computer technology. Doctors can no longer control their own disciplining, and medical associations must become public bodies governed in the interest of the public.

Emergency Services

Community emergency response systems should include properly designed, staffed and equipped ambulances and a communications system which means proper assistance will reach the sick and injured without delay. When practical, police cars should be converted into station-wagon-type ambulances. Helicopters also have an obvious role to play in transporting victims from crowded freeways and rural areas. Centralized computer banks should contain the case histories of each citizen, so that attending personnel lose no time. Emergency units and operating theatres in hospitals and clinics must be staffed and equipped in such a way as to assure minimum delays and red tape together with maximum efficiency and expertise.

The Role of Doctors and Nurses

What about doctors? In their hands lie so many of the answers to current problems and the responsibility to resolve them. Maybe they will remain the "captains of the team," but what other modern teams pay their captains ten to twenty times as much as the other players?

Doctors must also learn to play their part in controlling costs. In many cases prepaid group practice may be the answer. If doctors continue to refuse to play a part bringing costs under control, there is little hope for immediate improvement.

Tomorrow's nurse also has an increasingly important role to play. She must take over part of the work load of the disappearing general practitioner as she takes on more community responsibilities. She should also return to a closer association and contact with the patient.

However, if we can accept the need for the introduction of scientific management techniques, it is quite possible that the greatest manpower need in medical care is not for doctors, or nurses, or therapists, but rather for management personnel trained in hospital and business administration. If doctors wish to continue running hospitals let them take a hospital administration course, otherwise they should stick to doctoring. No longer should we permit doctors to run the "non-system." The "hoax" of doctor supremacy must be broken.

Medical Schools

Our Medical Schools must not only produce *more* doctors – but should also admit an increased number of students from geographic areas, economic backgrounds and ethnic groups, now inadequately represented. Medical teaching must be dovetailed with large mass movements in technical research and in social change. The future doctor must be trained with other workers on the team. As health science centres are encouraged to develop University affiliations, doctors should be trained with the other workers as part of a team. Medical education must be devoted to the health and medical care needs of the people. More public health and preventative medicine should be taught in our schools. Finally, our Medical Schools will have to graduate an increased number of general practitioners and primary care physicians.

150

Medical Research

Ottawa's and Washington's on-again-off-again approach to medical research has to cease if we are to stop the declining morale within the North American Medical Scientific community. Both Canada and the United States must redefine and update meaningful medical research policies. The Medical Scientific community should present realistic goals to the public if it expects to receive public support. More scientists will have to be trained in a host of associated disciplines, and far more of our scientific achievements must result much more quickly in better services and treatment for people at every level of society.

Public Health

Public health and preventative medicine must in future receive much more emphasis, both within and without our hospitals, and universities. This should involve more regular check-ups; an honest attack on pollution and environmental programmes; more effective powers for the Food and Drug Agencies on both sides of the border as we begin to pay greater attention to nutrition, and to the side-effects of drugs. Cleaning up the air in North America is the single most important thing we could do in the area of preventative medicine for the average urban dweller. Automobile and highways deaths and injuries must now be considered as an epidemic, a public health scandal, and be treated as such. Ottawa and Washington should set up National Accident Prevention Research Centres for accidents of all kinds. Federal authorities must truly improve methods for recalling defectively-built cars. Federal safety performance standards should ascertain that safety is really engineered into vehicles at the manufacturing level. The states, provinces and municipalities should begin to enforce laws, police and educate better and safer drivers, build better and safer roads. Regular and meaningful inspection of vehicles, together with a proper safety certification for second-hand cars before resale is another "must." The slaughter of the mechanized age *can* be stopped, as can the massive invasion of our environment. But it can be stopped only if we change our priorities and make a serious attempt to combat the diseases of affluence.

151

Preventative medicine must include much greater concern regarding questions of mental health. Not only do we need more psychiatric facilities and personnel, psychiatrists must also learn to incorporate their findings regarding human development into the process of social planning and change. This involves, for example, a knowledge of welfare programmes and housing conditions. Mental illness or breakdown should be recognized for what it is.

The Role of Industry

Industry, too, has a key role to play. The industrial revolution, and the benefits conferred by its assembly line and mass production techniques, speaks for itself. Yet, some of its side effects can no longer be tolerated by a society which chooses to call itself civilized and humane. Government regulation is surely only part of the answer. The original genius which was present in the industrial sector is still there, but too many spokesmen for industry automatically resist change and turn a deaf ear to contemporary interests and modern concerns. Contemporary thinkers, young and old, are turning their backs on past values, on a mass production system which uncritically devours valuable natural resources, and is based on controlled and planned obsolescence. Better living conditions, guarantees that products are "as safe as possible," are only part of the challenge. Industry spokesmen lose all credibility when they say they cannot meet it. If they can't, they should get out and make way for those who can. We can no longer wait.

Where Do We Go From Here?

Lack of public concern and interest is largely responsible for the present mess. Certainly an integral part in any advance necessitates enlightened public interest and action. As the shroud of mystery is lifted from medical activities, questions must be asked and performance demanded. In many ways this is already happening as a result of the information explosion which has taken place in our post-industrial society. Electric communications, in general, and television in particular, have brought out and exposed so many modern "problems" to public scrutiny. But the danger lies in the fact that everything we hear, see, or read about seems to be a "crisis" until we virtually become "crisis" immune, and we can no longer distinguish between *bona fide* and imaginary problems. It seems as if, all at once, every problem ever known to man has, simultaneously, been dumped in our laps for an immediate solution.

It is clear that we have confused our priorities; we have devoted a great deal of effort to the production of material goods and little effort to the care of the people who produce them. We have rushed ahead with cars, roads, factories, new food technology, without really knowing where we are going. Or why.

As a critic of medical and health care services in North America I say our health care services are in appalling disarray. We have been faced with real problems, a multitude of them, and we have thrown up our hands in despair.

Our society suffers from deep social wounds. Yet our approach is to put band-aids on them. We are only tinkering with the parts of the "non-system" and that is worse than nothing. We need major surgery.

Sources

The sources for a book such as this are many and varied. Primarily I conducted scores of interviews with people involved in medical and health-care services. Specific research projects were carried out by university students only too willing to help. I also attempted, when possible, to witness at first hand the scenes and conditions described in this book. Many associations in the medical and health-care field, and related areas, made their libraries available to me, as did universities. Through the kindness and help accorded me, I had a small library at my disposal by the time my basic research was completed.

The U.S. Information Service office in Ottawa was of great assistance. Clippings from American and Canadian daily newspapers, weeklies, and other periodicals for the years 1969-1971 were invaluable, as were the Canadian Press files on medical and health-care services, 1960-1970.

There were a number of basic sources for the book. They were: the *Proceedings* of the White House Conference on Health (1965); the *Federal Role in Health Report* of the U.S. Senate Committee on Government Operations (1970); the *Full Report* of Ontario's Committee on the Healing Arts (1970); the *Task Force Reports* on the cost of health and medical-care services in Canada (1969); the *Health Insurance Report* of Quebec's Commission of Inquiry on Health and Social Welfare (1967); the conference manuscripts of the Canadian Medical Association's sessions on medical insurance and manpower (1969); various papers delivered at the O.M.A.'s 90th Annual Meeting (1970); M. W. Griffith's *Health Care for All Americans (1970); Paul De Kruif's The Fight for Life* (1934); and David A. Baxendale's *Productivity in the Hospital Sector* (1969), which, while having particular application to the sections on hospitals, is also a valuable general source.

Sources for specific chapters or areas of concern follow.

Introduction

Rashi Fein's "Crisis in Our Medical Services" (in *Challenge*); Carroll Quigley's *The World Since 1939: A History* (1968); the *Report* of the U.S. National Advisory Commission on Health Manpower (1967); John Kenneth Galbraith's *The New Industrial State* (1968).

Emergency Services

Ontario Emergency Services Division's *Course Training Standards: Fundamentals of Casualty Care for Ambulance Attendants* (1970); *Report* of the International Conference on the Medical Aspects of Traffic Accidents (1955); Margaret Jones' Paper on Police Emergency Services; *Proceedings* of the U.S. Head Injury Conference (1966); *Proceedings* of the S.T.A.P.P. Conference (1955).

Dr. Harold Elliott (of Como, Quebec) and N. H. McNally (Director of the Emergency Services Division of the Ontario Hospital Services Commission) made available to me a great amount of material. Dr. Robert Kennedy's work as Director of the American College of Surgeon's Committee on Trauma was also invaluable.

Discipline and Control

Center for the Study of Responsive Law's *One Life, One Physician: An Inquiry into the Medical Profession's Performance in Self-Regulation* (1971).

Medical Manpower: Paramedicals, Education and Research

Report of the International Meeting of Group Medicine (1970); J. A. MacFarlane's *Medical Education in Canada* (1964); J. Wendell MacLeod's *Medicine's Responsibility to Society* (1970); J. R. Allen's *Appalachian Student Health Project* (1969); *Report No. 2* of the Medical Research Council of Canada (1968); the National League for Nursing and the Regional Councils and States Leagues for Nursing's *Action in Hospital Nursing* (1964); the Canadian Nurses' Association's *Report on the Project for the Evaluation of the Quality of Nursing Service* (1966) and *Rules, Functions, and Educational Preparation for the Practice of Nursing* (1969); Diane Charter's "Task Force Report; Blueprint for Action in Nursing Service" (*The Canadian Hospital*; March, 1970); Helen Mussalem's "The Changing Role of the Nurse" (*American Journal of Nursing,* May, 1969).

Health Maintenance and Preventative Medicine

J. H. Dale's *Pollution, Property and Prices* (1968); the Citizens Advisory Committee on Environmental Quality's *Community Action for Environmental Quality* (1970); Ralph Nader's *Unsafe at Any Speed* (1965); J. S. Turner's *The Chemical Feast* (1970); the Canadian Government's *Food and Drug Consumer Handbook* (1969); the *Interim Report* of the Commission of Inquiry into the Non-Medical Use of Drugs (1970); the *Final Report* of the U.S. Task Force on Prescription Drugs (1969); the U.S. Department of Health, Education and Welfare's *Study of Drug Purchase Problems and Policies* (1966).

Hospitals

Michael Crichton's *Five Patients: The Hospital Explained* (1970).

Costs

Final Report of the Special Committee of the House of Commons on Drug Costs and Prices (1967).

Quackery

J. H. Young's *The Medical Messiahs* (1967); Ian Collins' Paper on Regulation of Near Medicine, (1970).

Index

Brazeau, Dr. Paul, 120
Brière, Michel, 8-9
British Army, Medical Corps,
9
British Association for the
Advancement of Science,
125
British Medical Association,
132
Bronchial ailments, 122-123
Brose, Dr. Richard A., 16

Cabot, Dr. R. C., 28
Caloric need, 116
Calories, 116
Canadian Association of
Medical Colleges, 50
Canadian Breweries, 117
Canadian Council of Hospital
Accreditation, 74
Canadian Medical Association,
16, 28, 42, 94, 117, 132,
142, 144
Canadian Pacific Railway, 5
Cancer, 1, 37, 38, 63, 123,
131, 134, 144; of breast,
144; of cervix 113; of
colon, 114; of lung, 122;
pap smear test, 113; of
rectum, 114
Cappen, Dr. A., 120
Cardioratory, 65, 66
Cardiovascular, 61, 116
Carnegie Foundation, 48
Carnegie-Mellen School of
Industries Administration,
122
Carver Memorial Hospital, 84
Cass, Dr. Elie, 13

Castonguay Report, 54, 72,
77, 86
Catalepsy, 133
Centre for the Study of
Responsive Law, 24, 26
C. C. F. (Saskatchewan), 146
Charcot, Jean-Martin, 132
Check-up, 113, 128
Chief of Medical Staff, 97
Chief of Surgical Staff, 97
Chiropractor, 134
Cholera, 114
Cholesterol content, 116
Church of Christ Scientist,
134-136
Church of Scientology, 136-
137
Churchill, Winston, 121
Civil War, 25
Clark, Dr. Ronald C., 26
Clinical Investigation Unit, 67
Cobalt sulphate, 117-118
Cobalt therapy, 90
Code of Medical Ethics, 144
Cold, the common, 117
College of Family Physicians
of Canada, 34
College of Physicians and
Surgeons (Ontario), 25
College of Physicians and
Surgeons (Quebec), 29
Collin, Johanne, 29
Collip, 56
Columbia Presbyterian
Medical Centre (New
York), 11
Columbia University
Department of Nursing, 70
Commercial insurers, 102
Committee on Professional
Hospital Activities, 73

Elliott, Dr. Harold, 17
Emergency: care of the sick
    and injured, 16-17;
    standards for emergency
    department in hospitals, 17;
    standards for emergency
    ambulance services, 17
Emergency Health Services
    (Ontario), 9-10
Emergency Measures
    Organization, 21
Emergency Services Branch
    (Ontario), 9-10, 20
E-meter, 134, 137
Encephalitis, 115
English, Wilfred, 29
Enovid, 120
Estimates Committee of the
    House of Commons
    (Canada), 93
Evans, Dr. John, 58
Exercise, 116; programmes,
    116

Facilitators, 139
Faith Healing, 134-136
Family Health workers, 38,
    148
Federal Health programmes,
    46-47
Federal Safety Performance
    Standards (Canada), 151
Federman, Dr. Daniel, 43
Fein, Rashi, 104
Financial mechanism, 104-105,
    146-147
Financial reporting, 90, 148
Finch, Robert E., 118
Fleet, Dr. Thomas, 134
Fluoroscope treatment, 29

Flexner, Abraham, 48
Flying Doctor Service
    (Australia), 34
Folsom, Marian, 59
Food and Drug
    Administration (U.S.), 116,
    118-120, 138, 151
Fortune magazine, 105
Fragmentary billing, 105
Framingham Heart Study, 61
French Academy of Medicine,
    132
Fuchs, Victor R., 102
Funeral Directors, 8

Gabelein, A. C., 136
Galbraith, John Kenneth, 99
Gardner, Dr. Campbell, 8
General Accounting Office
    (U.S.), 84
Genetic engineering, 1
Generic name drugs, 109
German Measles, 115
Gilbert, Gloria, 70
Gillanders, Dr. Henry, 31
Goldbloom, Dr. Victor, 77
G.R.A.S. List, 118
Group Insurance policies, 103
Group practice, 44, 45, 47,
    105-106
Grove, J. W., 27
Guindon, Jean, 33

Hadacol, 138, 139
Hallucinations, 135
Hamelin, Georges, 32

Montreal General Hospital, 8, 17

Montreal Health Department, 36

Montreal Neurological Institute, 8, 55, 59

Montreal Police Ambulance Service, 19

Montreal *Star*, 77

Morgan, Mrs. Carolyn, 120

Morin, Dr. Y. L., 117, 118

Mortality rates, 2, 3, 9

Mount Sinai Hospital, 3, 29

Mount Zion Hospital, 3

Nader, Ralph, 121

National Academy of Science— Food Committee (U.S.), 118

National Accident Prevention Research Centres, 127, 151

National Congress in Medical Quackery, 131

National Health Service, (U.K.), 145

National Health systems, 146

National Institute of Health (U.S.), 46, 60, 61, 119

National Institute of Mental Health, (U.S.), 126

Navy (U.S.), 84

Neurolinometer, 131

New Republic, 99

New York Times, 26

Nightingale, Florence, 142

Nitrogen oxides, 123

North American medical schools, 43, 49

Nutrition, 116, 119

Obesity, 116, 133

Occult healers, 132

Occupational therapists, 68

Office of Economic Opportunity (U.S.), 84

Ogilvy, Richard, 18

Old people's homes, 86

Ontario College of Physicians and Surgeons, 27

Ontario Department of University Affairs, 133

Ontario Medical Association, 13

Open heart surgery, 86

Orwell, George, 91

Oscillators, 131

Oscilloclast, 131

Osler, Sir William, 56

Paetow, Dr. Paul E., 17

Painless childbirth, 135

Paramedical personnel, 41, 66, 67

Paraplegia, 8

Patent medicines, 138

Pathological laboratories, 75

Pathologists, 76, 105

Patient-focused nursing care, 89

Peckham, Justice, 130

Peer Review, 29-30, 78, 149

Pellerin, Dr. Richard, 31

Penfield, Dr. Wilder, 8, 55

Pentecostal, 136

Perkins, Dr. Elisha, 129

Perrault, Raymond, 9

Personality disorders, 143

Pesthouses, 79

Pharmaceutical manufacturers, 111
Philathea College (London, Ont.), 133
Phlebitis, 120
Physical fitness training, 115
Polio, 114, 115
Poverty, 111, 124, 130
Pre-operative preparation, 68
Prepaid group practice, 105, 150
Prescribed drugs, 111
Preventive Medicine, 79, 84, 91, 113, 116, 128, 148, 151, 153
Preventive psychiatry, 126
Primary care physicians, 150
Private, proprietary hospitals, 73
Proctological examination, 114
Provincial Department of Transport (Ontario), 21
Psychiatric hospitals, 89
Public Accounts Committee (Canada), 106-107
Public Health doctor, 113
Public Health Psychiatry, 126

Quaile, Basil, 103
Quebec College of Pharmacists, 110
Quebec Federation of Medical Specialists, 35
Quebec Health Department, 76
Queen's University: Medical School, 15-16; Department of Medical Studies, 27
Quigley, Carroll, 2

Radioclasts, 131
Raudin, Dr. I. S., 14
Rear Admiral, 93
Record keeping, 28, 30, 45
Regional and community clinics, 35, 39, 82-83, 148-149
Regional Hospital Planning, 81, 148-149
Rehovat, Israel, 140
Resuscitation rooms, 7
Roberts, Oral, 136
Rockefeller University, 46
Rice, Dr. Don, 34
Robb, Dr. Preston, 59, 63
Robillard, Dr. Raymond, 35
Rogerson, Carol and George, 12
Roy, Judge Paul Emile, 12
Royal Edward Chest Hospital (Montreal), 86
Royal Victoria Hospital (Montreal), 12, 107
Rural Ambulance Service, 35

Safety Certification for Second-Hand Cars, 151
Saint Mathias Anglican Church (Toronto), 136
Sarrazin, Michel, 56
Scientific American, 131
Scott, Dr. Charles, 120
Searle, G. D. and Co., 120
Secretary of Transport (U.S.), 22
Segal, Dr. Leo, 31
Self-care, 68
Self-dosage, 129
Self-hypnosis, 135

University of Kansas School of
    Medicine, 16
University of Manitoba, 57
University of Minnesota, 120
University of Montreal, 36, 61
University of Sherbrooke, 120
University of Toronto, 37
University of Utah, 120
Unrestricted Common
    property, 124

Vaccination Assistance Act
    (U.S.), 115
Varicose veins, 115
Vascular disease, 115
Viruses, 115
Voluntary hospitals, 79-81

Wall Street Journal, 110
Wardrope, Douglas, 14
Water-borne disease, 124
Weekend Magazine, 32
Weizmann Institute of Science,
    140
Whooping Cough, 114-115
Wilbur, Dr. Richard S., 39
Wise, Dr. Harold B., 37-39
Workmen's Compensation
    Board (Ontario), 135
World Health Organization, 37
World Medical Association, 28

X-ray, 7, 13, 38, 45, 80, 86,
    105, 107, 134

Yellow fever, 114
Youmans, Dr. Roger L., 16